Discover the Eye

Vince Zingaro, O.D.

Illustrations by Gregory DiNapoli

First published by Dog Ear Publishing
4010 W. 86th Street, Ste H
Indianapolis, IN 46268
www.dogearpublishing.net

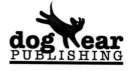

ISBN: 978-1-4575-1266-7

This book is printed on acid-free paper.

Printed in the United States of America

To Tammy

Table of Contents

ANATOMY OF THE EYE

W e don't think too much about our
eyes. To many people, the eyes are
just gelatinous spheres in our head that passively
filter light, allowing us to navigate our world. In
fact, they are much more than that. There are
many parts of the eye that cooperate to allow us
to interpret the world around us. Our eyes are
actually an extension of our brain. Before we can
understand the role our eyes play in our every-
day life, it is helpful to know some basic anatomy
of the eye and how each part works. We'll start
from the front of the eye and explain the major
parts and how they function to help us see.

The **eyelids** are extensions of the skin that
provide protection to the eye. We also rely on
our eyelids to help spread our tears evenly
across the eyes. When our eyes become too dry,
the eyelids have a difficult time performing this

duty, causing us discomfort and sometimes blurry vision. It would be similar to driving your car in a rainstorm with poor windshield wipers. Dry eyes that are uncomfortable should be evaluated by your eye doctor so that he or she can recommend an appropriate treatment regimen. This is often a complicated condition that can have many different causes, such as inflammatory conditions, dehydration and even the weather.

A twitching sensation of the eyelids is not at all uncommon. With the average adult getting less than seven hours of sleep a night, it's no wonder that we're feeling aches in our muscles and general fatigue throughout the day. Typically, adults should be getting somewhere between eight and nine hours of sleep each night. The same soreness that arises in the muscles of our back and legs can also express itself in the muscles of our eyes. Many people experience fatigue when the eyelid begins to twitch.

An eyelid twitch, or ocular myokemia, occurs primarily when the muscles of the eye become fatigued. The muscle then begins to spasm, causing a fluttering sensation around the eye. This condition may come and go throughout the day and may last from a few seconds to minutes. It's almost always harmless, however; the biggest worry that most folks have is the embarrassment that others may notice the eyelid twitching. Generally, most of your friends will never notice, as the movement is too small.

The best treatment for an eyelid twitch is easy: rest. Simply catching up on some much needed sleep is often the best remedy. If you're not quite ready to call out of work, then a gentle massage of the lid may calm the muscle. Aside from lack of sleep, other factors, such as caffeine, smoking, and stress, can contribute to this eyelid flutter, too. If you feel like you're getting enough sleep, consider minimizing these other factors as well. Maybe it's time for a vacation!

The eyelashes extend from the base of the eyelids. Eyelashes have two main functions: protection and positioning. They prevent debris and dust from entering the eyes. Not only does this keep the eyes comfortable, but it helps our vision, too. If we had dust and debris accumulating in our eyes, then we would have scratches on our eyes to the point where it would blur our vision. The same happens when we get scratches on the lenses of our glasses – the vision becomes distorted. Eyelashes also act as a sensor to let us know when an object is getting too close to the eye. When an object brushes against the lashes, the eyelids quickly shut to protect the eye. This is a protection mechanism similar to whiskers on cats. This can be a difficult reflex to overcome for someone who is new to contact lenses.

In the area near where the eyelashes meet the eyelids there are about 25 to 30 meibomian glands. These glands secrete an oily, fatty liquid that is responsible for making up part of the tear film that covers the eyes. Without this layer, the tears would simply evaporate into the air, leaving the eyes dry and the vision blurry. Occasionally, these glands can become clogged from dead skin, debris or inflammatory conditions. When this happens we have what most people call a stye. Sometimes these styes can be tender to the touch, but they almost always form a red pea-sized bump along the eyelids. We have bacteria that naturally call our eyelids home and don't cause us much harm. When these bacteria make their way into a meibomian gland, they can be the source of great discomfort. In this case, it is necessary to take an antibiotic to fight off this infection. In the majority of cases, however, simple warm compresses on the eye will usually clear out a stye (or a chalazion as your eye doctor may refer to it) in a few days.

The **cornea** is a clear, dome-shaped tissue that surrounds the front of the **iris**, or colored part of the eye. The cornea is responsible for proper focusing of the light coming into the eye to view the world around us. The cornea's transparency is due to the orientation of the protein strands that make it up. These thin, collagen fibers lie parallel to each other in a precise manner to allow light to easily pass through. There are no blood vessels in the cornea to provide oxygen and nutrients. The only way oxygen can reach the corneal tissue is through diffusion from the air. In fact, when we sleep, the cornea swells slightly because the eyelids cover it up and limit the supply of oxygen. The swelling recedes quickly after we awaken.

The **sclera** is the white part of the eye. It consists of a tough, protein tissue that wraps around the entire globe. Its two main functions are protection against trauma to the eye and prevention of light from entering the inside of the eye. The thickness and fibrous tissue of the sclera keeps the retina dark to allow for better image resolution. You can imagine how hard it would be to watch a movie in the theater if there were windows to allow light inside. In a similar way, the sclera ensures that our vision is sharp by providing a safe, dark environment.

Overlying the sclera is the **conjunctiva.** This very thin, translucent layer of tissue lines the sclera and inside half of the upper and lower eyelids. Inflammation of this layer can cause conjunctivitis, or pink eye. Conjunctivitis literally means inflammation of the conjunctiva. Conjunctivitis can occur from bacteria, viruses or from an allergic reaction. Depending on the variety of conjunctivitis it can also be very contagious, so it is important to seek treatment sooner rather than later to avoid spreading the condition to others.

As we move further back through the eye, we arrive next at the **iris** and **pupil**. The iris is the colored part of the eye that regulates the size of the dark hole in its center, the pupil. When we step outside on a bright sunny morning in the summer, light passes through the pupil into the eye. When this happens, signals from the brain are sent to the iris to make the pupil as small as possible because too much light will cause the image in the eyes to be blurry. Likewise, when we enter a dark movie theater there is relatively little light that is passing through our eyes. In this case, signals from the brain are sent to the iris to make the pupil as large as possible to allow more light into the eye. In both of these instances, the goal is to allow the proper amount of light into the eye to gain the optimum resolution of the world around us.

As we know, iris color varies greatly around the world. Genetics dictates whether we will have light blue eyes, dark brown eyes or anything in between. Parents with very dark eyes tend to have children with a similar color. The actual color is determined by how much pigment is present in the iris. The more pigment, the darker the eyes look. Most of the time eye color resembles skin and hair color. A man from Germany with blonde hair and fair skin is much more likely to have blue eyes than a woman from Zimbabwe with dark skin and dark hair. A darkly pigmented iris is usually dominant over a lightly pigment iris. For example, children of a mother with very light blue eyes and a father with very dark brown eyes tend to have an eye color more closely resembling their father.

In front of the iris and behind the cornea is an open space filled with a clear fluid called the anterior chamber. The fluid present in this space is called aqueous humor. Its purpose is to physically support the cornea by providing a pressure against it. It also contains cells that support the immune system in and around the eye. This aqueous humor circulates through the pupil so that it reaches the anterior chamber and posterior chamber of the eye. The aqueous humor is produced in the eye and it drains out of the eye through a filter in the anterior chamber, leaving through the bloodstream. This filter is called the trabecular meshwork. Problems encountered in this area can put people at risk for glaucoma, which we'll discuss in detail later.

As we travel through the pupil into the posterior chamber, we immediately locate the magnifying glass-like structure called the **lens**. The lens consists of a collagen protein similar to the material in the cornea. It is about the size and shape of an M&M, although rather than being filled with chocolate it is completely clear and surrounded by a clear shell. Over time, this clear inner area of the lens becomes a cloudy yellow color. When this happens, it is called a cataract. Cataracts will be discussed in more detail later.

The main function of the lens is similar to the cornea in that it focuses the light passing through our eyes into a sharp image. It does this in conjunction with the ciliary muscle that is attached to both sides of the lens. The ciliary muscle is unlike our biceps that allow us to lift with our arms. While we can easily flex our biceps, we do not have conscious control of our ciliary muscles. These muscles contract and relax depending on how clear or blurry an object is that we are looking at. When we focus on an object in the distance, such as a bird nesting in the top of a tall tree, the ciliary muscles relax the tension on the lens. This causes the lens to straighten out flat. As you are reading this book, your ciliary muscles are contracting to bend your lens in precisely the correct position for you to read these words. The more the lens bends, the closer we can hold an object in focus. To understand this, imagine if you picked up a paper plate and held it at three o'clock and nine o'clock, and slightly pulled both sides toward you. Your hands would be the ciliary muscle and the paper plate would be the lens. Over the course of our life the lens becomes less bendable and though the ciliary muscles are still as strong as they have ever been, the lens can not bend into the correct position to help us see objects close to our face. This condition will be discussed in greater detail later.

Behind the lens is a gel-like substance called the **vitreous** body. The vitreous is clear to allow the light penetrating the eye to pass without distortion. Like many other clear parts of the eye, it is made up of a collagen protein that is thin enough so that light can pass through, allowing us to see. The main function of the vitreous is to support the retina both physically and nutritionally. You can think of the vitreous as having the viscosity of maple syrup, except it is clear. It has a different consistency depending on our age. In children, the vitreous is almost 100% gel. Over time though, the protein that holds this gel together begins to break down. When this happens, the vitreous changes from a thicker gel to a more liquid form. As this process occurs, pieces of the gel can break away from the rest and float around the eye. Many people describe these "floaters" as bugs, cobwebs, hair, string – you name it. What is actually being seen are the tiny pieces of the vitreous body that are floating around in the back of the eye. Floaters can usually best be seen when one looks up at the sky on a clear day or against a plain background, such as a white wall.

For the most part, vitreous floaters are harmless. On occasion a rather large section of the vitreous breaks apart and suspends itself in the center of the eye, causing a spot that doesn't seem to move. This is called a posterior vitreous detachment (PVD). Nearly everyone over the age of 65 years will experience this in at least one eye. A PVD can put you at risk for a retinal detachment. To be safe, if you notice any spots in your vision, be sure to have them examined by your eye doctor as soon as possible.

The last main structure of the globe of the eye is the **retina**. The retina is the part of the eye onto which light is focused and an image is formed. It consists of many different cell types, however we'll focus on two of the more common and important ones – the rods and cones.

There are approximately 96 million rods and cones in the retina. Rods are responsible for allowing us to see in low light situations. When we're trying to find the best seat in a dark movie theater, rods are doing all of the work. They are specialized to allow us to see in dim light, however they do not allow for crisp, clear vision. Most of the rod cells are located in the outer portion of the retina. This allows them to contribute to our peripheral vision. Without them, we would lose a bit of our sense of space. Our peripheral vision allows us to avoid running into people in a crowded mall during the holidays and increases our ability to drive safely along a busy highway. There are many more rod cells in the eyes than cone cells, as the rod cells are more uniformly distributed in the retina.

In contrast to the rods, there are relatively few cone cells. The cones are almost entirely all located in a special area of the retina called the macula. The macula is the part of the retina where the image is formed from the light that gets reflected off of an object. Fortunately, our cones are located here, because they allow for color vision and fine detail in our vision. The main reason we're able to see clearer when looking straight ahead rather than off to our periphery is because most of the cones are located in the macula, which is the center of the retina. Any problems affecting the area in and around the macula will cause big problems for our vision. We'll get into more details about what can go wrong here later.

From the retina we exit the back of the eye along the **optic nerve**. This structure is extremely important, as it is the connection between the eyes and the brain. All of the information from the retina is sent along this nerve which heads to the back area of the brain, the occipital lobe. This connection is interesting, because as the optic nerve enters the retina from the brain it branches off into millions of nerve fibers, which suggests that the eyes are really an extension of our brain.

The point in the retina where the optic nerve enters creates a blind spot in our vision. This is an area in the retina where there are no rod or cone cells. The reason why we don't walk around with two dark spots in our vision is that our brain amazingly fills in this spot with our environment. To better grasp this phenomenon, try finding your own blind spot using the figure below. Cover your right eye and look directly at the cross, holding the page approximately 18 inches away from your face. Slowly move the page closer and you will notice that at some point the face will completely disappear. Keep moving it still closer and it will re-appear again. It may seem like magic, but the face disappears because our brain is filling in the face with its surroundings, which in this case is the rest of the page.

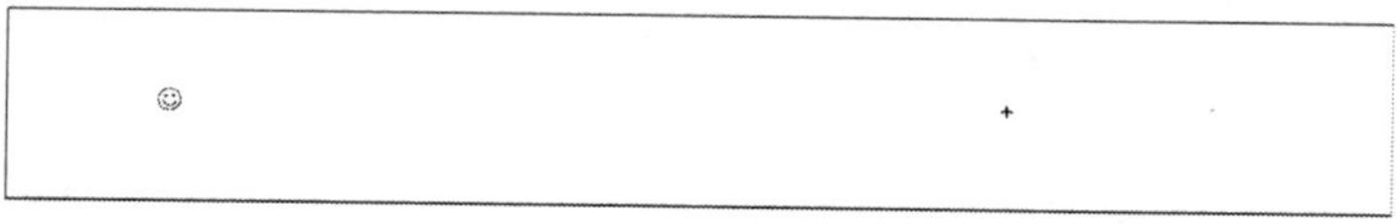

Figure 1.

As you can imagine, anything that affects the health of the optic nerve can cause serious problems with our eyesight. We'll examine several diseases that can affect the nerve later. The eye's close relation with the brain explains why many vision problems can arise after traumatic injury to the head. A jarring tackle in football or a severe automobile accident, among other injuries, can cause us to experience blurry vision, double vision and loss of vision. Any damage to the brain can have a ripple effect through all of its parts, including the eyes.

NEAR SIGHTED, FAR SIGHTED, AND EVERYTHING IN BETWEEN

How we perceive the world around us is almost entirely tied to our vision. In the majority of polls asking people which of the five senses they feel is most important, the sense of sight is almost always valued most. Our sense of sight is in constant use from deciding which groceries on the shelf at the market we should purchase to keeping our balance. (Try standing on one leg with your eyes open versus your eyes closed; it's much more difficult without the use of your eyes.) Our eyes tell us when we're in danger and help us to know when we're in love. Since nearly everyone's vision is different, it is interesting to see how various vision anomalies affect our lives.

Many of us enjoy hearing from the eye doctor that our vision is 20/20, even though many of us don't fully understand what it means. It just sounds good. The top number in the ratio (20/20) is the number of feet between an object and a person. It is almost always 20. The bottom number of the ratio is roughly the distance in feet that someone with what we would call "normal vision" would be able to stand to see the same object that you are viewing. For example, let's say you and a friend are looking at the letter "E" on a street sign. You are standing 20 feet away from the sign and can clearly discern the letter "E" on the sign while your friend (who incidentally has normal vision) can stand 100 feet away from the sign and still clearly see the letter "E". Your vision in this case would be 20/100. You should probably make an appointment for an eye examination. On the other hand, if you can stand 20 feet away and see the letter "E" on the sign while your friend has to move up to 15 feet to be able to see the same letter, then your vision would be 20/15, quite impressive! This is simplified a bit, but you can now appreciate how your vision is categorized at your next eye examination.

According to the American Optometric Association (AOA), about 30 percent of the population in the United States has myopia, or near-sightedness. Someone is considered near-sighted when they can see objects up close clearly, but cannot see objects at a distance. The degree of near-sightedness or far-sightedness is measured in units called Diopters (D). The extent of how far a nearsighted person can see an object in the distance is dependent on how many Diopters of myopia is present in their eyes. Someone with only one Diopter of myopia in each eye can still see everything around them relatively clear for about 5 to 10 feet before the world begins to get blurry. Someone with 9 D of myopia cannot see an object much more than a few inches away from their eyes.

There are two main reasons that myopia can occur. The first is that the eye is too long. The average length of the eye is about 24mm. It only takes a few extra millimeters of length to cause a moderate amount of myopia. When the eye is longer than average, light entering the eye through the pupil is focused in front of the retina rather than exactly on the retina. The result is the same as if the focus was off on a camera. This is perceived as a blurry image.

The second reason that myopia can occur is that the cornea has too steep of a curve to its shape. If the clear, dome-shaped cornea is too long, then light passing through it will be focused too far in front of the retina, causing an object to appear blurry. This is the most common reason for someone to be nearsighted.

There is a strong belief among scientists that myopia is hereditary. Like most areas of genetics, however, it is not as simple as it may sound. It is thought that myopia is inherited with a 50-80% variance. This means that about half or slightly more of our myopia comes from our mother or father and the rest comes from our environment.

Scientists sometimes group childhood myopia separately from adult onset myopia. Most cases of myopia occur during childhood and teenage years. When we are nearsighted at a very young age our level of nearsightedness tends to be greater than adulthood. It is thought that the environment contributes more to nearsightedness for those who require glasses or contacts to see far away at age 29, for example. It turns out that our eyes were not exactly designed to be staring at a computer for nine hours a day, five to six days a week.

Farsightedness, or hyperopia, is not as straightforward as one would think. By definition, being farsighted means that objects in the distance can be seen clearly while near objects are somewhat blurry. The catch here is that people less than 40 years of age can usually see far away and up close very clearly with up to almost 2 D of hyperopia. To understand how this can happen, we need to think about what happens in the eye of someone who has hyperopia.

When someone is farsighted, the light reflected off of an object passes through the pupil and comes to a focus behind the retina. This is the opposite of what happens in myopia. The main reason for this is the shape of the cornea. If it is too flat or not curved enough, then the light gets focused too far behind the retina. This causes an object to appear blurry. In general, people with hyperopia tend to have smaller eyes, typically less than 24mm.

What is interesting about farsightedness is that the lens can make up for a small amount of blurry vision. As I mentioned before, typically the lens is in a flat position when viewing an object in the distance. If an eye happens to be farsighted, however, looking at this object will appear blurry, because the image will be in focus behind our retina. When this happens, the brain almost instantly signals to the ciliary muscle to bend the lens to help bring the object into focus. This bending of the lens causes the object to come into focus precisely on the retina instead of behind it. This will work for small amounts of hyperopia, however an eye with 6 D of hyperopia, for example, will still have difficulty focusing on an object in the distance. Regardless, if our ciliary muscle and lens have to work this hard all day there is a tendency to get what some people describe as eye strain or "tired eyes" by the end of the day.

The ability to see through a small amount of hyperopia does not last forever. In fact, people with hyperopia typically notice a decrease in their distance vision in their mid-forties. This happens because the lens in the eye becomes less flexible over time and is unable to bend as easily as in a younger person. This process occurs gradually over time and those who are farsighted typically need some sort of glasses or contact lens correction to bring their vision back to where it was 20 years earlier.

People with hyperopia are not the only ones dealing with a changing lens. In fact, around the age of 40 is when the phenomenon of presbyopia occurs. Presbyopia comes from the Greek word *presbys*, which means "old man". It is an experience that we will all have eventually as the lens becomes less flexible. This rigidity of the lens makes it difficult to see clearly up close. Going back to our paper plate analogy, in presbyopia the paper plate has now become a ceramic plate. Even though the ciliary muscle, our hands in this case, has roughly the same strength as it did twenty years ago, the lens is no longer pliable enough to bend into the position that we need it to for clear vision.

The process of presbyopia occurs in everyone, but its effects are different depending on whether you have myopia, hyperopia, or no prescription at all. For those who have myopia, the annoyance of presbyopia can be overcome by simply removing the glasses or contacts that are worn for distance viewing. The person with 2 D of myopia means they have 2 D of "near sight". In this case, 2 D of myopia would allow a person to see clearly close up without any glasses or contact lenses until they reach their mid to late fifties. For the person who has 2 D of hyperopia, however, the scenario is quite different. In this case, since they will already need an extra 2 D of "near power" when they reach presbyopia, they will have greater difficulty viewing a book, menu or cell phone. Many times, these folks can be seen holding items such as these further away from their face to make them clearer. This allows for a more comfortable viewing position, because the further away an object is viewed, the less the lens needs to bend to properly keep the object in focus. Since we can't grow our arms any longer, presbyopia often warrants the need for bifocals.

To many people, the word "bifocal" is as bad as some other four-letter words we may know. In fact, the word bifocal has two parts: "bi" meaning two and "focal" referring to focus points – one for distance and one for near. That's it. Bifocals do not imply that someone is legally blind or that now someone has to wear the same style of glasses that her grandmother did. Nor do bifocals imply anything about the thickness of the glasses. They certainly should not invoke the image of "Coke bottle" glasses that some folks can remember having many years ago. Having only been in practice a relatively short amount of time, I am amazed at the different meanings that patients have devised for the word.

There are bifocal glasses, trifocal glasses, progressive glasses and even bifocal contact lenses. They all function to treat presbyopia. Progressive lenses have become increasingly popular in recent years for a couple reasons. First, they look better cosmetically because there is not a visible line in the lens that we see in other multifocal glasses. Second, since they progressively increase in power from the top half of the lens to the bottom half of the lens, there is an infinite range of vision depending on which part of the lens one looks through. A drawback to this type of multifocal lens, however, is that there is some peripheral distortion when looking out the sides of the glasses because of the physics involved with not having a line in the lens. A number of patients have the complaint that they simply have to turn their heads up and down too much to get decent vision. Regardless, there are many different options for those of us who struggle to see far away and close up. We will discuss vision correction options in more detail later.

We shouldn't end this chapter without discussing another obstacle that can stand in the way of visualizing the world around us. Astigmatism is present in most eyes. Astigmatism occurs when the cornea or the lens of the eye is not shaped properly. This irregular physical shape causes the light that is reflected off an object to become focused at many different points on the retina instead of one point. The result is blurry or distorted vision. To understand this, imagine a basketball sliced in half. When you look at one half you get a perfectly spherical half dome of the basketball. This is how a cornea with no astigmatism would look; completely round with no stretching or oval shape to it. If you took the same basketball half and pulled on opposite ends at twelve o'clock and six o'clock, you have now changed the shape of the basketball. The opposite ends (three o'clock and nine o'clock) have begun to move closer together. The basketball would nearly resemble a football at this point. This is what a cornea with astigmatism looks like. Since the cornea is no longer a perfect sphere, the light coming through the cornea into the eye gets distorted. The analogy is a bit of an exaggeration, but you get the point.

Astigmatism is thought to be hereditary, although scientists are not fully certain. In fact, there are probably numerous factors that play a role in determining how much astigmatism will be present in one's eyes. There is a large amount of research being done on a condition called keratoconus, which leads to very high amounts of astigmatism in the eye.

Keratoconus is a condition that causes a progressive thinning of the cornea. This gradual thinning causes the cornea to take on the shape of a cone. As we have seen before, anything that causes a drastic change in the shape of the cornea from its half basketball shape will cause big problems with the vision. In fact, people suffering from keratoconus experience extremely distorted vision and especially have trouble with glare. Driving at night, even while wearing glasses or contacts, is often impossible. The distortion is often so great that people will note seeing two or three images at once. Aside from the visual problems of keratoconus, some folks become sensitive to light and have pain and discomfort in the eye.

It is estimated that about one in 2,000 people worldwide have keratoconus. Although the

exact cause of keratoconus is still poorly under-
stood, there are a couple of leading theories on
its existence. A hereditary basis is thought to play
some role. It is estimated that less than 25% of
patients with keratoconus also have a family
member with the disease. A second theory on
the cause of this condition is that allergies could
be a larger contributor than we may think. People diagnosed with keratoconus show a higher
percentage of allergies than the general public.
The thought is that allergies cause the eyes to
itch and thus we rub them. Rubbing of the eyes
over time can physically alter the delicate tissue
of the cornea, causing distortion. If this theory
has any merit, it may allow us to treat keratoconus before any major symptoms are present.

The current management of keratoconus
primarily involves the use of contact lenses. In
mild cases, it is sometimes enough to properly
correct one's vision with a simple glasses prescription that will correct for the astigmatism.
Eventually, the disease progresses enough where
the vision is usually not quite good enough with
glasses. When this happens, the next step is to
attempt to fit the individual with contact lenses.
With mild to moderate keratoconus a soft contact lens is often enough to achieve adequate
vision, however rigid contact lenses frequently
work better with higher amounts of astigmatism.

When attempts to correct vision in people
with keratoconus fail with glasses and contact
lenses, we are left with a surgical alternative. A

corneal transplant is necessary when the cornea becomes too hazy or so cone shaped that contact lenses cannot fit properly. A cornea is taken from an eye bank (yes, even our eyes are used when we sign up to be an organ donor!) and tested to be sure that it is a suitable match. This procedure has been performed for several decades with great success. Fortunately, surgery is only used as a last resort and is often not necessary unless a diagnosis of severe keratoconus has been made.

Hopefully you now have an appreciation of the various ways we view the world. There are many different perspectives courtesy of the small, intricate parts of the eyes and brain. If these nuances were the only barrier standing in our way of perfect vision, then my job would be a whole lot easier. It turns out there are a number of problems that can arise causing our sight to be blurry, distorted or lost forever. Let's now discuss some of the most remarkable, yet common troubles to affect the eyes.

CATARACTS

There are many misconceptions about what cataracts are, who gets them and how they occur in our eyes. To many people cataracts invoke an image of Grandma or Grandpa sitting in a rocking chair telling us stories of the Great Depression. While it is certainly true that the majority of people who have had cataract surgery are generally over 60 years of age, the truth is that cataracts can affect people of any age. A good understanding of what cataracts are and why they can cause vision problems is essential to being able to make educated decisions with your eye doctor about your treatment options. It is also important to understand the best ways to prevent cataracts from forming earlier than necessary.

A cataract is a clouding of the lens in our eye as a result of the breakdown of the proteins

within the lens. If you remember our lens as having an appearance similar to an M&M candy it is
easier to imagine exactly how a cataract forms.
The outer colored layer of the M&M resembles
the outer shell, or capsule, that surrounds the
lens, and the chocolate part of the candy would
be comparable to what we call the nuclear cortex of our lens. Instead of chocolate in our lens
we have a crystal-clear protein layer that is precisely arranged in an exact manner to allow light
to freely pass through. Over time, the metabolism
of the lens pushes the new material out from the
center of the lens to the outer regions in a circu-
lar fashion – similar to the rings of a tree. As this
happens, the older protein material in the center
begins to break down and lose its transparent
nature. This causes the formerly clear proteins to
turn slightly yellow in color. As we approach our
60's and 70's this process speeds up and our lens
goes from being clear as water to a yellow-
brownish looking color. Since it is no longer clear,
light entering our eye cannot reach our retina,
which distorts our vision. Another good analogy
here would be to imagine a dirty window that
hasn't been cleaned for ten years. Dust, dirt and
debris build up on the window and we are no
longer able to see through it as we once did
when it was brand new. The same process occurs
in our eyes. The lens becomes dirty or cloudy
over time, which causes our vision to become
impaired. When our lens gets cloudy enough (or

ripe, as some doctors refer to it) surgery is necessary to remove the lens and replace it.

There are three main kinds of cataracts. The most common type is called a nuclear sclerotic cataract. In this case the nuclear cortex in the center of the lens becomes increasingly cloudy and develops a yellow color such that over time it distorts our vision. When we talk about cataracts developing in older folks, we are generally referring to this sort of cataract. A less common type of cataract is a cortical cataract. Unlike nuclear sclerotic cataracts, these tend to form from the outside of the lens and grow toward the center. Doctors often call this "spoking" as these cataracts resemble the spokes of a bicycle wheel. They are not necessarily as yellow as the more common nuclear sclerotic cataracts, but they have distinctly defined edges. Finally, another less common form of cataract is called a subcapsular cataract. These form on the lens capsule itself and not on the inner part of the lens (the candy coated shell of our M&M, not the chocolate part). Because of their position on the central part of the capsule, these cataracts tend to cause more problems with daytime viewing than nighttime viewing. In the daytime our pupils tend to be smaller, whereas in the evening the light is dimmer and our pupils are larger to allow more light to pass through. Therefore, this particular cataract blocks more of our vision in the daytime when our pupils are smaller. People who have this type of cataract also tend to notice more problems with their near vision – reading, knitting, and working at a computer – than with their distance vision. A subcapsular cataract is more commonly found in people under the age of 65, because these cataracts are typically the result of a traumatic injury to the eye or a systemic disease that affects the body, such as diabetes. They can also result from taking certain medications, such as steroids, for a prolonged amount of time.

There are many different causes of cataracts. The most common reason for having cataracts is simply our age. The older we get, the more likely it is that our vision will be impaired by cataracts. Nearly everyone over the age of 65 has at least the beginning stage of cataracts. Unfortunately, our age is not something that we can control. The good news is that we *can* control many other frequent causes of cataracts. The cumulative effect of ultraviolet light from the sun over the course of our lifetime is known to accelerate cataract formation. This is one reason why it is important to wear sunglasses. Certain prescription medications, such as steroids, along with cigarette smoke, diabetes, and trauma to the eye round out the list of the top reasons for cataract development. All of these causes disrupt the delicate proteins that make up the lens. Even minuscule changes to these proteins can increase the risk of cataract development.

We have known about cataracts since the ancient times. The current English word for cataract comes from the Arabic term meaning "waterfall", because the vision of someone with cataracts was often described as though one was looking through a wall of water. About 2,500 years ago it was thought that cataracts were the result of an evil liquid that formed in the eyes and caused blindness. Anatomical studies of the eyes of animals eventually led to the discovery that in fact cataracts were an opaqueness of the lens. The earliest form of cataract treatment was called couching and involved the use of a needle to penetrate the cornea and simply move the cataract out of the way. You can imagine this feels about as good as it sounds – terrible! Fortunately for us, technology has greatly improved this procedure for the better. The couching method has been eliminated and we now simply take the cataracts out of the eye. The cloudy lens is removed and replaced with a crystal clear plastic lens.

It's important to realize the enormous impact that cataracts have on our vision worldwide. Cataracts are the leading cause of blindness in the world. There are nearly seven billion people on Earth and about 45 million are blind. In medical terms, when we say people are blind it means that their vision is worse than 20/400. In other words, they can't see past three or four inches from their face. Some of you who are very nearsighted can imagine that your life would be very different if you did not have accessibility to eye care that provides glasses or contact lenses. Most people in this group of 45 million people are elderly or come from developing countries. The biggest reason why these folks cannot see properly, however, is because they have cataracts in their eyes and have no access to proper eye care. Fortunately, there are wonderful organizations, such as the Lions Club International, that sponsor humanitarian missions to developing countries to provide much needed care.

There are a couple reasons to undergo cataract surgery. The main reason for surgery is because our quality of life in our day-to-day activities becomes diminished due to poor vision. Remember, glasses and contact lenses can only correct our vision to a certain point. It doesn't matter how sharp the image is coming into our eye, if it has to pass through a cloudy window we are simply not going to see well enough. This is the time to consider having cataract surgery. Many doctors will refer to cataracts as being "ripe", meaning that the cataract has matured enough and is causing a decrease in the quality of a patient's life to the point where it is reasonable to have surgery. A second reason to have cataract surgery is out of medical necessity. Sometimes, the cataract can become too ripe, or hypermature, and the lens begins to swell to a point where it can block the drain where the aqueous humor leaves the eye. This can cause an unsafe rise in the pressure in our eye, since aqueous humor continues to be produced at the same rate, but drains at a much slower rate. Removal of the cataract helps to unclog the drain. Not only can a cataract block the drain, but it can sometimes progress so much that the proteins begin to leak out of the capsule of the lens. Our body identifies these proteins as foreign particles, because it has never had direct contact with them. The immune system starts to attack the foreign particles. This can cause quite an inflammatory reaction, which will cause the eye to become painful and irritated. People who are farsighted (hyperopia) are more likely to have the cataracts removed for medical reasons, since they have smaller eyes for the cataracts to cut off the aqueous humor drainage.

The process of undergoing cataract surgery is pretty standard. After a thorough eye examination, your doctor will calculate the exact power of the new lens that will take the place of your cloudy lens. Most of the time blood work is necessary to ensure that you are healthy enough to undergo the surgical procedure. A few days before the surgery, your eye doctor will have you take eye drops to prevent infection and inflammation. These drops are critical to allow the eye to heal properly and for the vision to reach its maximum potential. In most cases, the patient is awake during the surgery, although a sedative is usually given to decrease any discomfort or anxiety that may occur. The eye itself is completely numb during the entire operation. There is a common anxiety among people that they might accidentally blink during the operation, but fear not! During the surgery your eyelids are held open by a lid speculum which will not allow you to blink. Of course your eyes are numb, so you experience no pain at all.

The latest and greatest form of cataract surgery involves a procedure called phacoemulsification. First, the surgeon makes two small incisions just a few millimeters wide along the edge of the cornea. This allows for the insertion of a small instrument that is thinner than the diameter of a pen to penetrate the cornea to have access to the lens. The instrument slides through the incision and creates a small hole in the front capsule of the lens. This is necessary to get to the inner cortex of the lens so that we can remove the cloudy material. Once the surgeon has gained access to the cortex of the lens, the next step is to break this hard, lumpy material into smaller, more manageable pieces. This is accomplished with the use of an ultrasound instrument that moves through the second incision created in the cornea. The ultrasound tool is about as thick as a needle and uses sound waves to crush the hard cataract into smaller pieces. This is why your eye care provider may send you for surgery sooner rather than later, because if the cataract has become too ripe it becomes a bit more difficult to break up with the ultrasound device. In general, the more mature the cataract becomes, the more effort we must use with the ultrasound to smash the cataract up into smaller pieces. Once we break down the cataract, we simply use a suction device to clean out the cloudy material.

It's almost like using a vacuum (although a very expensive one) to sweep away the debris. Throughout this procedure saline fluid is pumped into the lens area of the eye to maintain the support of the lens and cornea. Now that we have a hollowed out lens capsule it is time to insert our new artificial lens. Since we are dealing with an opening only a few millimeters wide, the new lens is folded in half and carefully placed through the corneal incision and into the lens capsule. Once the new lens gets into the capsule, it gently unfolds and is manipulated by the surgeon to the correct position. Phacoemulsification is wonderful, because it typically doesn't require the use of stitches to heal such a small incision in the cornea. The whole surgery is painless and takes about 30 minutes to perform for a routine case.

After cataract surgery, patients must be seen for follow-up appointments at one day, one week, one month and three months from the day of the surgery. The eye drops that are taken prior to the surgery are continued for at least a month from the surgery date. The follow-up appointments and eye drops are necessary so that the eye can properly heal from the surgery and the maximum vision potential can be realized. The anti-inflammatory drops ensure that swelling does not develop in the retina. Fortunately, this is not a common occurrence. You will also be required to wear an eye shield at bedtime for about a week to protect you from inadvertently rubbing your eyes in your sleep. Your eye doctor also wants to make sure that a retinal detachment has not occurred. Although this is rare, a retinal detachment occurs when the retina begins to peel away from the back of the eye. We generally wait about two weeks before removing a cataract in the other eye if it is needed. The two-week waiting period ensures that your eyes and body have fully recovered from the trauma of the first surgery. It is also advisable not to do any heavy lifting or strenuous activity for several weeks after the procedure. Exactly when sports and physical activity can be resumed are at the discretion of the eye doctor.

Cataracts cannot form again once they are removed, but the formation of "secondary cataracts" is fairly common. These are not actual cataracts (they cannot be, since we have completely removed the lens of the eye), but rather connective tissue that accumulates around the new lens and causes cloudy vision. This is called a posterior capsular opacification. Only about one in four people who have cataract surgery will experience symptoms of decreased vision and noting halos around lights. Fortunately, this is easily corrected with a laser treatment that only takes a few minutes. The laser blasts the connective tissue away from the new lens giving a new window for clear vision. This laser procedure is only necessary once, if at all, after cataract surgery.

The best way to slow the development of cataracts is to maintain a healthy lifestyle. Quitting cigarette smoking now can significantly cut your risk of needing early cataract surgery (aside from increasing your health in every other part of your body). Wearing sunglasses is another way to prevent cataracts. It is especially important to wear sunglasses when you are near water or snow. The reflective surface of the water and snow increases the intensity of the sun's rays, causing further harm to your eyes. Ultraviolet light from the sun is thought to cause cataracts in a similar way that it can cause skin cancer. As the light passes through the lens of the eye, it causes the formation of free-radicals or unstable molecules that cause damage to surrounding molecules, proteins and DNA in the body. These free-radicals cause the proteins of the lens to break down, eventually leading to cataract formation. There have been mixed results as to the effectiveness of beta-carotene, vitamin E and niacin to prevent cataracts. These anti-oxidants help prevent free-radical formation. Leafy-green vegetables that are high in vitamins and anti-oxidants are great to incorporate into your diet to not only improve the health of your eyes, but also to improve the overall health of your body. A good multi-vitamin might be all that is necessary for you, but be sure to check with your doctor.

Before we wrap up our cataract chapter, let's briefly discuss congenital cataracts. By definition, these cataracts are present at birth. They are often found in newborns with other genetic diseases, but they can also be present in an otherwise healthy baby. This type of cataract is usually inherited from the mother or father. They can occur in one or both of the eyes. Babies that have congenital cataracts have leukocoria (white pupil), as the doctor can usually detect the cataract by shining a light into the pupil. When these cataracts are detected, surgery is usually done as soon as possible, especially if there are cataracts in both eyes. The reason for this is to prevent future vision loss. If the newborn child does not have enough visual stimulation, then the eyes and brain cannot develop the proper nerve connections to allow for good vision. After cataract surgery, the child is carefully monitored for any loss of vision. Many times glasses or even special contact lenses are necessary at a very young age for the child to enjoy adequate vision. It is thought that the rate of congenital cataracts is much higher in developing countries, where the impact is much greater because of the lack of eye care.

As we have noted earlier, cataracts continue to be the leading cause of blindness worldwide. Fortunately, today's standards for cataract surgery are outstanding and the outcome has been extremely successful. I've had many patients who were thrilled that they no longer needed glasses to see in the distance after cataract surgery. It is important for people in countries without adequate access to cataract surgery to limit the risk factors that cause cataracts. Through public awareness and mildly altering our lifestyle, we can hope to minimize the effects cataracts have on our way of life in our country and around the world.

GLAUCOMA

Like cataracts, glaucoma is an often misunderstood disease. Some people use the term cataracts and glaucoma interchangeably. In fact, glaucoma is a dangerous disease of the eye that can permanently take away our vision. You can develop glaucoma if you are young or old. I have seen firsthand the devastating vision loss that this disease can render in folks who simply thought that their glasses or contact lens prescription needed an adjustment. The difficult aspect in the detection of glaucoma is that, for the most part, it is a gradual, painless loss of vision over time. Unlike a toothache, the eye can suffer irreparable damage without any warning signs until it is too late. Glaucoma's stealth nature is the reason why eye doctors always check for early warning signs during a comprehensive eye examination and also highlights the importance of having your eyes checked annually.

Glaucoma can be defined as progressive damage to the optic nerve that results in vision loss. Peripheral vision is usually affected first, followed by a gradual destructive path toward our central vision. It is generally a slow moving disease that causes vision loss over a period of years rather than days or weeks. It will eventually cause blindness if left untreated. While it is not exactly certain what causes this damage to the optic nerve, it is known that an elevated pressure in the eye can play a key role in vision loss from glaucoma. An increased pressure in the eye is not, however, necessary for a diagnosis of glaucoma.

According to the World Health Organization, glaucoma is the second leading cause of blindness on Earth. In the U.S. alone, nearly 2.25 million people have been diagnosed with glaucoma. These numbers by themselves are high, but what is troubling is that there are millions more people who probably have glaucoma or are at a high risk for developing glaucoma who do not know it, because they have never had their eyes examined. Glaucoma can occur at any age for the most part, but it more commonly affects our vision beginning around 60 years of age. Since it can take 10 to 30 years to cause damage, your eye doctor will almost always check your eyes for signs of glaucoma during your comprehensive eye examination.

There are a few different forms of glaucoma, but the most prevalent type is called primary open angle glaucoma (POAG). The angle here refers to the "drain" (trabecular meshwork) discussed earlier, which is responsible for filtering the fluid (the aqueous) out of the eye and back into the bloodstream. When the angle is open it means that at least some of the aqueous in our eye is able to leave. The pressure of the eye will increase when either too much aqueous is being produced or not enough aqueous is being drained. In essence, glaucoma is somewhat of a plumbing problem. In POAG, the pressure is too high inside the globe of the eye, exerting a damaging force on the optic nerve. This nerve, like any other nerve in our body, is very sensitive to its surroundings, so an abnormal eye pressure can cause damage resulting in vision loss over time. The pressure that we are referring to here only relates to the force of the fluid being produced in our eyes, not our blood pressure. This is a common misconception. Blood pressure can play a very minimal role in affecting our eye pressure, but only when it reaches dangerously high levels. Typically, POAG is responsible for around 75% of all forms of glaucoma. Since this is the type of glaucoma most commonly encountered in the general population, I will be referring to POAG whenever glaucoma is mentioned in this book. We will discuss other types of glaucoma at the end of this chapter.

As an eye doctor, I can tell you that making a diagnosis of glaucoma is a bit like solving a puzzle. There is no one specific test that tells us definitively if someone has glaucoma. We have to gather and analyze data from several different tests and procedures to determine the best plan of action. The most common parameter that is needed is the intraocular pressure in the globe of the eye. A normal pressure measurement is anywhere between 10mmHg and 20mmHg. If we could say that anyone with a pressure above 20mmHg had glaucoma, it would make my job much easier. Unfortunately, some people can have a pressure of 25mmHg and be completely healthy, while others may have a pressure of 14mmHg and have a substantial amount of vision loss. The complex role of eye pressure adds to the mystery of glaucoma.

There are two ways to measure the pressure in the eye. First, we could use a non-contact tonometer that blows a strong blast of air onto your cornea and gives us an indication of the pressure by how much air must be used to exert a certain force on the eye. This method is not quite as accurate (or as comfortable) as the second method used to determine eye pressure: Goldman tonometry. When we use a Goldman tonometer, the doctor will instill a yellow drop in the eye which contains a fluorescent dye and an anesthetic. The dye allows the doctor to see your eye better under the slit lamp. The anesthetic gently numbs your eyes so the doctor can use a small device that contacts the front surface of your cornea to determine the pressure. This method is the gold standard in measuring eye pressure and it is used in most eye care practices. Both methods determine the pressure by analyzing how much force it takes to indent a certain area of the cornea. These procedures are similar to those used for determining how much air is in your bicycle tires. If you can push in rather easily on the tire or squeeze it, then you assume the tire pressure is low and you need to fill it with more air. On the other hand, if you can't really push much on the bicycle tires, then you can safely assume that the pressure is high enough that you wouldn't need to add any more air.

Another piece of the puzzle in deciding whether one has glaucoma or not is determining the thickness of the cornea. If we think about our bicycle tire analogy we can understand the importance of this test. Imagine two bicycle tires, one that is very light and built for racing in the Tour de France while the other is very heavy and built for riding across dirt and rocks. The smaller, lighter tire may be quite easy to push because it is very thin. We can easily squeeze the tire in our hands even if it has a substantial pressure. The larger, heavier tire will not be quite as easy to squeeze in our hands because it is very thick. We would have to squeeze the thicker tire much harder than a thinner tire of equal pressure. When a cornea is much thicker than normal, we have to push a bit harder on it. This causes our pressure readings to be a bit higher in an eye with a thicker cornea than it would be in an eye with a thinner cornea. If we can determine the corneal thickness, then we can have a better idea of the accuracy of the pressure reading in our eye.

Gonioscopy is a procedure that is done to examine the structures of the angle. Blunt trauma to the eye, whether from a hard punch to the face or a line-drive off of a baseball bat, can severely damage the delicate angle of the eye. If this occurs, there is the potential for the pressure in the eye to build up, which can lead to glaucoma. A gonioscopic lens is placed on the eye and allows the doctor to indirectly view the angle to assess any damage. The narrower the angle, the slower the aqueous leaves the eye, which causes an increase in the pressure. It is imperative to make sure the drain is open for the aqueous to properly flow out of the eye.

One of many things that eye doctors examine when dilating the pupils is the optic nerve. When looking for glaucoma this is one of the most important parts of the exam, because the doctor is able to get a three-dimensional view with his or her own eyes at the optic nerve. A cup to disc ratio is often analyzed to get an idea of how much healthy tissue remains of the optic nerve. The cup of the optic nerve is an area where there are no nerve fibers leading back to the brain. The disc is the area of healthy nerve fibers that transmit information from the retina to the brain. The cup to disc ratio is the area where the space of absent nerve fibers is compared to the remaining healthy nerve fibers. A cup to disc ratio of about .4 is normal. This means that 40% of the nerve fibers leading to the brain are absent. The ratio varies among different races and age, but typically a cup to disc ratio around .7 will generally raise a red flag for glaucoma. People of African descent typically have a larger cup to disc ratio than Caucasians. If the cup to disc ratio increases over time, it indicates that nerve fibers are dying. This important figure is nearly always noted when a dilated eye exam is done, regardless of whether or not doctors suspect that someone has glaucoma.

If there are enough warning signs that someone may have glaucoma, eye doctors often run two other tests to help confirm their suspicions. First, a visual field test will be needed. This test assesses a patient's peripheral visual field and compares it to a database of "normal" peripheral visual fields. This test checks for any detectable vision loss from glaucoma. Second, it is important to have a laser scan of the optic nerve to quantify exactly how much healthy tissue is present. The laser creates a three-dimensional picture of the optic nerve allowing doctors to track changes in the appearance and depth of the nerve over several years. This test is usually repeated annually so that immediate action can be taken if any changes are noted. There are several different laser devices on the market that differ in operation; however, they all give us similar results to analyze the integrity of the optic nerve.

Once we have all of the pieces of the puzzle, doctors can use this data to make a diagnosis. The decision to treat glaucoma is based on all of your data and genetics. There have been several studies suggesting that the risk of glaucoma increases in those people who have family members with the disease. As with other conditions that may be inherited, it seems most relevant to compare immediate family members only. Your uncle or cousin who may have glaucoma may not influence your doctor's decision to treat you as much as if your mother or father may have suffered from the disease. If your doctor feels that your risk of developing glaucoma is too great, he or she will initiate treatment. Vision cannot be restored once it is gone, so the idea is to prevent further vision loss in a patient.

The general treatment goal for glaucoma is to lower the pressure in the eye. Currently, this is the only way that is known to slow the disease from progressing. The main theory is that lowering the pressure in the eye will reduce the physical stress on the optic nerve. A common goal to aim for is a 30% reduction in the eye pressure. Studies have revealed this to be adequate for halting the progression of glaucoma. The current eye drops on the market work in one of two ways. First, there are drops that will decrease the output of aqueous fluid production.

Alternatively, there are drops that can increase the rate of the aqueous exiting the eye. A more recent group of drops that are quickly becoming the standard for glaucoma treatment are the prostaglandins. These drops work by increasing the output of the aqueous leaving the eye. The prostaglandins combine the greatest reduction of intraocular pressure with the convenience of only one drop per day dosing. The less we have to use drops during the day, the more likely we are to remember to take them.

For the most part, the use of eye drops is sufficient to stop many cases of glaucoma from getting worse. On occasion, different classes of drops must be used together to get a maximal effect. For example, we may prescribe a prostaglandin drop with a drop that also decreases the rate of aqueous fluid production. If the eye drops are not bringing the pressure down to an acceptable level, then the next step is a procedure called selective laser trabeculo-plasty, or SLT. Here, a laser is used to target specific pigmented cells in the trabecular meshwork, the filter that allows the aqueous fluid to drain from our eye. When these cells are targeted by the laser, debris from the cells is scattered within the trabecular meshwork. This action triggers the immune system to bring in cells called macrophages to clean out the debris and allow the fluid to flow more easily through the trabecular meshwork. The advantage of an SLT is that it is painless and can be repeated several times if the pressure needs to be lowered again. Sometimes, the pressure is low enough after a SLT that eye drops are no longer necessary. The length of time that the procedure is effective varies from a few months to a few years. For people with glaucoma, the SLT is a valuable tool to reduce the pressure where eye drops have failed.

When drops and laser treatments aren't enough, surgery is the last resort to stop glaucoma. Remember, the only way doctors can stop glaucoma is to keep the pressure in the eye at or below a target goal. In some cases there are people who are on maximum treatment with drops and laser management, but still face eye pressures that are too high and are causing their glaucoma to progress. A surgical procedure called a trabeculectomy creates additional space in the trabecular meshwork by removing pieces of it for the aqueous fluid to flow through. A series of tubes are inserted to redirect the outflowing fluid, subsequently lowering the pressure. It is possible to bring the pressure down to around 5mmHg, if necessary. This procedure is very effective, but surgery is usually saved as a last resort because of the inherent risk involved. In some cases, a trabeculectomy can actually make the pressure in the eye dangerously low. A pressure of less than 5mmHg has the potential to collapse the anterior chamber of the eye, which can do further damage. As with all the treatment options in glaucoma, doctors are only able to stop the disease from causing further damage.

We currently cannot restore vision that has already been lost.

Although primary open angle glaucoma is the most common form of the disease, it is worth noting that several other types of glaucoma do exist. In normal tension glaucoma, there is optic nerve damage with a relatively "normal" intraocular pressure. The word "normal" here is used carefully, because there really is no normal pressure. The pressure may be around 15mmHg, but if there is optic nerve damage it must be treated in the same way as POAG – by lowering the pressure. In pigment dispersion syndrome, pigment from the back of the iris rubs off and becomes scattered about the eye. These pigment particles have the potential to clog the trabecular meshwork, which causes the aqueous fluid levels to build up and create a high eye pressure. If the pressure becomes elevated in pigment dispersion syndrome it turns into pigmentary glaucoma. This condition is more common in people under the age of 40, and in many cases will resolve with time.

I have been asked several times by patients about the effects of marijuana on the eyes. It is a common perception that once a diagnosis of glaucoma is made, it is time to head to the doctor for some medical marijuana. While it is true that marijuana can moderately decrease the pressure in the eye, doctors never use it as a treatment for glaucoma for the simple reason that there are better drugs on the market to achieve an optimal level of eye pressure. In the early 1970's, it was first discovered that marijuana could lower the pressure in the eye, but not necessarily low enough to prevent further damage of the optic nerve from glaucoma. The levels needed to accomplish this were so great that the side effects of marijuana outweighed the benefits. Since then, the idea that smoking marijuana cigarettes can be used to treat glaucoma has been put to rest.

Glaucoma, as we have seen, can be a very devastating disease that is complicated by the fact that not everyone responds to treatment in the same way. Some patients respond really well with one drop, while others require multiple treatment regimens to get the same effect. There is also debate among eye care providers as to exactly when treatment should be initiated. An old standard of care was to wait until there were signs of damage to the optic nerve that were revealed on the visual field test. If there was no damage, then there was no need to treat. This idea has changed somewhat recently, as research has revealed that by the time discrepancies on a visual field test show up, much more damage has already occurred than originally thought. Today, a more aggressive approach has been taken by many eye doctors to avoid such losses. For as many people who have actually been diagnosed with glaucoma, there are many more who we classify as glaucoma "suspects." These patients are

carefully monitored, sometimes more frequently than other patients, because of the
potential for them to develop glaucoma. Exactly
what makes someone a glaucoma suspect
depends on how many warning signs are
revealed on our numerous tests to rule out glaucoma. For the most part, when glaucoma is
caught early enough, most people who are com-
pliant with taking their drops and following up
with their doctor's recommendations won't lose
any further vision. The destructive nature of the
disease is the reason why doctors screen for
signs of glaucoma at each annual eye exam.

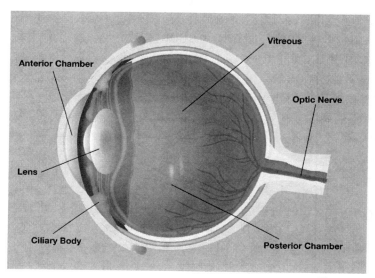

Figure 2

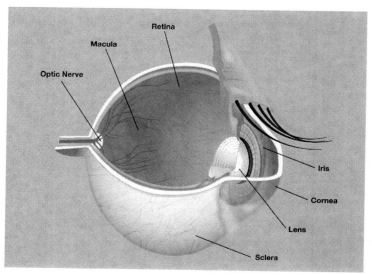

Figure 3

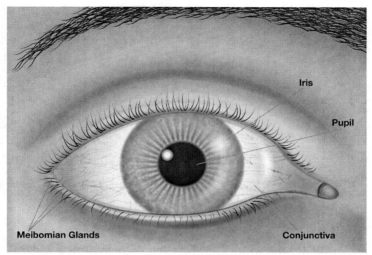

Figure 4

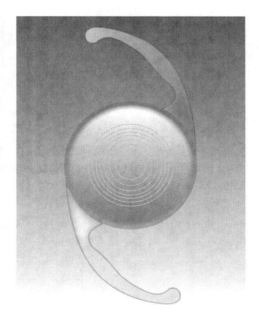

Intraocular Lens

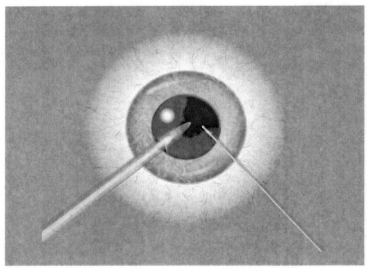

Phacoemulsification

MACULAR DEGENERATION

Over the last twenty-five to thirty years the average life expectancy around the world has gradually increased as medical technology and awareness of a healthy lifestyle have improved. People are living longer, healthier lives and there has been a steady increase in the number of folks who make it to 100 years of age. As we age, our risk of disease generally increases. There are numerous forms of cancer, for example, that are primarily seen in the over 70 population. Our eyes are no different than the rest of our bodies in this regard. Macular degeneration (MD) is an example of a disease that affects the elderly. Incidences of macular degeneration have been on the rise and show no signs of slowing down anytime soon. Research efforts aimed at finding a cure for this disease have intensified, since diagnoses of macular degeneration will skyrocket as the "baby boomer" generation becomes older. It's important to understand the causes, treatments, and most importantly ways this disease can be prevented from robbing people of their vision.

As discussed earlier, the macula is the area of the retina where the majority of cone cells are located. This is the area of the retina that is responsible for observing fine detail. Macular degeneration destroys the cells of the retina or, more specifically, the macula. The root cause of the disease is that cells in the macula begin to have trouble breaking down their cell waste products from their metabolism. As a result, the waste products build up to a toxic level that results in the death of the cell. As the cell dies the waste products that are remaining form discrete, yellow plaques that are called drusen. Similar to other parts of the body, the cells in the retina rely on their proximity to each other for communication, nutrients and general survival. As more and more drusen accumulate, it causes an enlarged space between the surrounding cells, which in turn places an increased stress on them. Eventually, this stress is enough to kill the cells.

Like any other cell in the body, the cone cells of the retina rely on blood transported though the arteries to provide oxygen. As the drusen levels build up in macular degeneration, it cuts the oxygen supply to the surrounding cells, because the blood vessels can't reach their destination as they did before. To compensate for this lack of oxygen, the blood vessels begin to form new branches that carry blood directly to the remaining cone cells in a process called neovascularization. This sounds like a great adaptation by the body to help nourish the cells; however, these new blood vessels are extremely fragile and will often break down, causing bleeding and scarring to occur. The process of neovascularization is actually very harmful to the retina and results in devastating vision loss. As we'll see shortly, stopping these new blood vessels from forming is part of the new treatments we're using to slow down the progression of macular degeneration.

The entire course of macular degeneration is one continuous process, but it is often defined as two separate entities: dry or wet. We classify the disease as dry macular degeneration with the detection of drusen in the macula. This is the first indication that the cells in the macula are not able to break down their waste products. At this stage the vision is not typically affected. Sometimes, people will develop only a drusen or two, but never fully progress to macular degeneration. When the disease does progress, there is an increase in the size and number of drusen. The dead cells can also produce pigmented areas that form around the drusen, which can potentially lead to vision loss. The impact of drusen on vision primarily depends on how large of an area they inhabit and how many of them form. As they invade a large enough area, people tend to notice a dark spot in the center of the vision. This spot is sometimes preceded by a distorted area of the vision that may cause objects to look larger, smaller, slanted or curved. In each case, however, this damage affects only the central vision where the cone cells of the macula reside. The "dry" prefix in this stage of macular degeneration indicates that there is no bleeding or scarring caused by the process of neovascularization. The majority of people (80-90%) who have been diagnosed with macular degeneration have the dry form.

As we discussed earlier, bleeding and scarring results as drusen build up to levels that disrupt the amount of oxygen reaching the macula. We describe wet macular degeneration as the point when the newly-formed blood vessels begin to bleed. At this stage, vision loss is usually significant. Depending on the size of the hemorrhage, vision can range from an extremely blurry 20/100 to only being able to perceive light. It is crucial to stop the bleeding as soon as possible due to the potential for scar tissue to form in the area of the hemorrhage. The longer the bleeding occurs, the greater chance that scar tissue will form and destroy what's left of the macula. Wet macular degeneration is obviously more debilitating than dry macular degeneration, but fortunately it is present in only 10-20% of those diagnosed with the disease. People who have been diagnosed with wet macular degeneration in one eye are at a significantly higher risk of developing the disease in the other eye.

Part of what makes this disease so destructive is that it affects the central vision. As the disease progresses through the end stages, people can be observed tilting their head slightly in order to use what peripheral vision they have left to look at something. It is difficult to imagine, but if you place your hand about one inch from your eye and close your other eye, you can get some sense as to how debilitating the disease can render one's vision. Once the entire central vision is destroyed, a person is left essentially blind in the eye.

Macular degeneration affects about 1.8 million people in the United States. It is the leading cause of blindness in people over the age of 70. While the exact cause of macular degeneration is unknown, there are risk factors that increase its prevalence. It is more prevalent in Caucasians, especially those with lightly colored eyes. We very rarely see this disease affecting black people, as they tend to have darker eyes with plenty of pigment to absorb harmful ultraviolet rays from the sun. This disease also tends to run in families. If your mother or father has been diagnosed with macular degeneration, then you are at an increased risk of developing the disease as you age. As the old name implies (age-related macular degeneration), we see most cases of this disease affecting people over the age of 65 years. This is perhaps the most important factor in acquiring the disease. People who smoke are also much more likely to develop macular degeneration as they age. There are some juvenile forms of macular degeneration, but these are exceptionally rare. For the purposes of this chapter, when I talk about macular degeneration, I'm talking about the more common form that primarily affects senior citizens.

Since there is no cure for macular degeneration, it is important to know all of the options to prevent the disease. In 2001, the National Institute of Health released a breakthrough study that showed the benefits of antioxidant vitamins and zinc in slowing down the progression of dry macular degeneration to wet macular degeneration. The report came from the Age-Related Eye Disease Study (AREDS) and states that supplementing the diet of patients diagnosed with early or intermediate stage macular degeneration reduced the risk of progressing to the advanced stage of the disease by approximately 25%. High doses of vitamin C and E, along with copper and zinc, were the key ingredients in decreasing the advancement of the disease. This was the first study that provided solid evidence of good nutrition as a factor in preventing the disease. It was previously known that diets high in leafy, green vegetables seemed to help prevent the onset of the disease; however, the antioxidants in the

AREDS formula are at levels that would be difficult to consume through diet alone.

The AREDS vitamins are widely available through several companies that produce a pill that is typically taken twice daily. Although the vitamins are available over the counter, it is important to note that they should not be taken without the consent of an eye doctor after a thorough dilated eye examination. These high dose vitamins can be harmful to smokers and can cause unwanted side effects, such as anemia, for non-smokers. The AREDS showed that these vitamins only reduce the risk of progression to advanced disease in people with mild to moderate forms of the disease. The AREDS vitamins have no ability to prevent or delay the development of macular degeneration in people who have not been diagnosed with the disease.

AREDS 2 is a follow-up study to the results released in 2001 that is researching the effects of lutein, zeaxanthin and fish oil in reducing the progression of macular degeneration from early to late stages of the disease. The results of AREDS 2 can be expected around 2013. Those currently at risk for wet macular degeneration are anxiously awaiting the final report from this exciting study. In the meantime, preliminary data from the study seem to indicate that lutein, zeaxanthin and fish oil will play a larger role in protecting the eyes from this blinding disease. It is important to note that this data is preliminary; we won't know exactly whether these added supplements will slow the progression of macular degeneration until the final data is analyzed and released.

Diet is one of the most important aspects of our life that will affect our well-being. Not only is a diet rich in vitamins and antioxidants good for overall health, but it can be a sight saver when it comes to macular degeneration as well. Diets high in leafy, green vegetables, such as spinach, kale and broccoli have been associated with lower rates of vision loss from macular degeneration. These vegetables contain plenty of vitamins A, C and E along with lutein and zeaxanthin. Incorporating a few of these foods into your diet can go a long way in ensuring the health of the eyes and the rest of the body.

While we want to consume plenty of vision saving antioxidants in our diet, we need to keep out harmful ultraviolet rays from the sun. There are three types of ultraviolet (UV) rays: UV-A, UV-B and UV-C. Most of the UV light emitted from the sun is UV-A. Exposure to excessive amounts of UV light is known to cause serious health problems. UV light damages our DNA, which is responsible for allowing regeneration of the cells of our body. The cumulative effect of UV light over a lifetime can disrupt the DNA of the cells in the macula. This malfunction of the macular cells leads to macular degeneration. It's best to make sure that you wear sunglasses when you're going to be outside in the sun for long periods of time. This is especially true when you find yourself sunbathing at the beach or skiing on the slopes on a sunny day. The water and snow reflect an even greater amount of harmful rays than usual in these scenarios.

Finally, the best lifestyle choice that you can make to avoid succumbing to macular degeneration is to stop smoking. I won't go into great detail about the harmful effects that smoking can cause the eyes (or every other part of the body), but I will tell you that quitting smoking can potentially add years to your life and your vision. If you smoke, you must stop immediately. If you need help with kicking the habit, contact your primary care doctor as soon as you can. You must do it now to save your vision and your life.

When preventative measures fail and wet macular degeneration develops, there are limited, but promising treatment options. Our treatment goal is to stop the development and bleeding of blood vessels caused by neovascularization. Traditionally, when we detect areas of neovascularization and bleeding in the macula we incorporate photodynamic therapy (PDT) as the main treatment selection. In this procedure a dye is injected into a patient's bloodstream that acts as a marker to show exactly where the "leak" is coming from in the macula. The dye is injected intravenously through the arm. It travels through all of the blood vessels of the body, including the leaky blood vessels in the eye. When viewed through a slit-lamp microscope, we're able to aim a laser at the vessel to seal off the bleeding.

Although photodynamic therapy has been adequate in eliminating neovascular blood vessel formation, the future may hold better treatments. PDT works well, but needs to be repeated when neovascularization occurs. It isn't a great long-term option for the treatment of wet macular degeneration. Doctors on the cutting edge of treating wet MD are using anti-VEGF (Vasoendothelial growth factor) drugs to stop the process of neovascularization. Anti-VEGF drugs were originally used in the treatment of certain types of cancer. VEGF is the chemical that signals the process of neovascularization to begin. Anti-VEGF drugs kill the chemical and in effect, stop new vessels from forming. In some cases, vision can actually improve. The drug is administered via injections through the sclera and into the retina (after a good anesthetic, of course). Currently, some anti-VEGF drugs are being used off label, but they have produced outstanding results so far and may be formally approved to treat wet MD in the very near future. This seems to be the best option to combat the devastating effects of wet MD.

As we now know, macular degeneration can be a debilitating disease that cannot only take away vision, but can also have an effect on the outlook of life for our elderly citizens. Someone who has gone completely blind in both eyes has the potential to become depressed. This is especially true of senior citizens who may not be able to be as physically active as they were in their younger days, and enjoy reading and other activities that are heavily dependent on their eyes. The best way to prevent MD and to ensure the well-being of your eyes is to have them examined each year by your eye care provider. This includes a dilated examination so that the retina can be carefully evaluated and signs of macular degeneration (and plenty of other conditions) can be detected as early as possible. If early MD is detected, the patient is often given an Amsler grid to take home and monitor for any changes in vision between eye examinations. It looks like a simple grid with a dot in the center, but it allows the patient to alert the doctor to changes when distortions are noted. As people are living longer lives, it is important to take care of ourselves so that we may live longer and *healthier* lives.

DIABETES & HIGH BLOOD PRESSURE

It seems appropriate to discuss diabetes and hypertension (high blood pressure) in the same chapter, because they both have similar effects on the eye. These diseases have the potential to cause blindness, are relatively common in our society and the number of people diagnosed with both diseases continues to rise. The American Diabetes Association reports that 18.8 million Americans have diabetes and there are roughly seven million people that probably have the disease, but have not been diagnosed. Nearly two out of three people with diabetes also have hypertension. The costs to treat these deadly diseases can be enormous. The damage that diabetes and hypertension can inflict on our bodies, including our eyes, is massive. Let's examine these conditions and see how they can impact our vision and our lives.

Diabetes is a disease in which there is too much sugar (glucose) in our blood. In the medical world, we refer to this as hyperglycemia. When we eat food, it gets digested and the nutrients are absorbed into the bloodstream to be distributed throughout the body. These nutrients, including sugars (in the form of carbohydrates), are used by our tissues for energy. As the sugar level rises in the bloodstream a signal is sent to the pancreas to produce a hormone called insulin and secrete it into the bloodstream. Insulin is responsible for transporting sugar in the bloodstream to the tissues of our body, such as our muscles. The amount of insulin produced is equal to the amount of sugar in the blood. For example, after a large Thanksgiving meal, our pancreas works very hard to secrete insulin to take the carbohydrates in our blood and distribute them to the tissues. As the sugar levels decrease, so does the amount of insulin secreted by the pancreas. A normal blood-glucose (sugar) level is around 70-130mg/dL. In diabetes, the blood-glucose level can reach five times the normal range. The root cause of diabetes revolves around insulin; either not enough of it is produced relative to the amount of sugar in the blood or the insulin molecule itself does not function properly. When either of those scenarios occur, the blood-glucose levels rise to a point that becomes dangerous to the body. As a result, the tissues do not receive the energy they need to keep their cells alive. Also, the blood itself can become sticky, resulting in blood clots, strokes and hemorrhaging. The damage is often irreversible and can lead to death.

There are two types of diabetes that are simply referred to as Type I and Type II. In Type I diabetes, there is a problem in the pancreas in that it does not produce enough insulin. There are many different names for this including "juvenile diabetes" and "insulin-dependent diabetes". Most people with this type of diabetes are diagnosed at a young age; usually under the age of 30 years. The quality of the insulin is fine; the problem lies in the insufficient quantity produced. For this reason, people with Type I diabetes are required to take insulin injections to regulate their blood-glucose level. It is often more difficult to control the blood-glucose levels in Type I diabetes because foods contain various amounts of sugar, which must be met with the proper amount of insulin. Type I diabetics can have more complications as they age because of the length of time with the disease and its effect on the kidneys. This form of diabetes tends to have a strong genetic factor associated with it as people become affected by the disease at a younger age than most Type II diabetics. This means that those people with a family history of diabetes must pay extra attention to their diet and amount of exercise to avoid development of the disease.

Type II diabetes is often referred to as "non-insulin dependent" or "adult-onset" diabetes.

These names can be misleading, because there are plenty of people with Type II diabetes that must use insulin injections to properly regulate their blood-glucose levels. In this form of the disease we generally have a problem with the quality of the insulin rather than the quantity, although we can have problems with both. When too much sugar is ingested in our body our pancreas can go into an "overload" mode. As food is constantly being broken down, insulin is constantly being produced to meet the demand for energy. The problem is that over time the receptors on tissues that are responsible for drawing in the insulin and sugar begin to break down from overuse. Since the insulin cannot deliver the sugar out of the bloodstream, it is rendered ineffective and the blood-glucose levels rise as a result. Many times the pancreas simply breaks down from working too hard. With a poor diet, the signal being sent to the pancreas to produce more insulin never gets shut off. Imagine if you set your air conditioner at a very low level and never adjusted it; you would probably be calling the repair technician sooner than you would like. The same scenario applies to the pancreas. If it is working too hard all the time it will eventually stop doing its job. At this point, simply controlling one's diet can produce dramatic results. Sometimes oral medications can be used to help restart the failing insulin and tissue receptors. If, however, the blood-glucose levels remain elevated, then the pancreas becomes affected and secretes less insulin. When this occurs, people with Type II diabetes will be required to take insulin injections to regulate the sugar level in the blood. Obesity, physical inactivity, and a poor diet are all to blame for the development of Type II diabetes, which is the most prevalent form of the disease. This emphasizes the importance of living a healthy lifestyle.

Although diabetes affects nearly every part of our body, the two main organs that are susceptible are the kidneys and the eyes. We have two kidneys in our body that are about the size of our hand and lie on each side of the spine of our lower back. Their job is to filter the waste from our body. Roughly 200 quarts of blood gets filtered each day through our kidneys, getting rid of nearly two quarts of waste products and excess water. These waste products are excreted out of our body in the form of urine. As you can imagine, without our kidneys we would not live very long due to the toxic waste products that accumulate in our body as a result of our metabolism. The kidneys are very robust and we can usually live quite well with only one functioning kidney. Diabetes harms the kidneys by damaging the filtering cells, called nephrons, as elevated blood-glucose levels wear down and eventually kill the nephrons. When enough nephrons die, the kidneys fail.

Kidney failure prompts the need for a kidney transplant. It can take a month or more to find a donor and set up the transplant surgery.

Sometimes people with kidney failure will need to undergo dialysis to rid the body of waste while they wait for a transplant. This involves connecting a dialysis machine to the body to remove, filter and replace the blood. Typically this needs to be done three days a week. As you can imagine, this can be an enormous inconvenience along with a substantial financial burden.

Before the kidneys have failed from diabetes, the eyes have usually suffered at least some of the harmful effects of the disease. Diabetes causes the small blood vessels of the eye to leak. The vessels of the retina that bring blood to nourish the optic nerve and the macula are particularly vulnerable to damage. When the blood-glucose levels reach unhealthy levels, the walls of the arteries and veins start to break down. This causes hemorrhaging along with fatty exudates (transported in the blood) to leak out into the retina and the vitreous. In a style similar to macular degeneration, this bleeding obstructs the vision and can lead to scarring. The more scarring that is present, the more likely there will be permanent vision loss. Bleeding and scarring in the retina also increase the chance of neovascularization from occurring. This creates a devastating cycle that results in eventual blindness.

Unlike macular degeneration, diabetes can attack all parts of the eyes. Remember, diabetes affects the blood vessels which perfuse our entire body. This is of importance in the eyes because diabetes disrupts the blood flow through the iris and anterior chamber, which brings an increased risk of neovascularization in these areas. The danger is that bleeding and scarring can clog the trabecular meshwork that is responsible for the aqueous outflow from the eye. When this happens, neovascular glaucoma can develop. This painful form of glaucoma is dangerous, because it can cause the pressure in the eye to spike very sharply in a relatively short amount of time. Optic nerve damage results at an accelerated rate. When neovascularization becomes so rampant in the eye that it leads to blindness and pain, there is often no other choice than to remove the eye. Thankfully, today's treatment options make this a rare scenario.

When diabetes affects the eye, damage is often first detected in the retina. Here, it causes "dot and blot" hemorrhages, so named because when doctors view them they look like drops of blood in various sizes and shapes. The medical term for this is called diabetic retinopathy. The longer someone lives with diabetes, the more likely he is to develop diabetic retinopathy even if the blood-glucose levels are kept at reasonable levels. Diabetic retinopathy is classified into three stages: mild, moderate and severe. As the disease progresses doctors stand on a high alert for neovascularization, which marks the beginning of proliferative diabetic retinopathy. At this stage doctors must take an aggressive approach to destroy the fragile, leaky blood vessels that have formed in order to prevent scarring and further vision loss. We use a special laser (Pan-Retinal Photocoagulation or PRP for short) that scatters around 1,000-2,000 small burns across the retina to halt the progression of neovascularization. Although, this method is painless, it can slightly diminish night vision and color vision. When proliferative diabetic retinopathy is present, laser treatment is almost always necessary to improve the vision in the eye.

Sometimes diabetes causes so much damage to the retina that the blood vessels begin to hemorrhage into the vitreous and throughout the globe of the eye. When this occurs, the hemorrhage makes it too difficult to aim a laser at the blood vessel to seal off the leaks, so we must resort to a procedure called a vitrectomy. As the name suggests, this procedure involves removing the blood-filled vitreous from the eye and replacing it with a saline fluid. This procedure is a bit more involved than laser treatment, but it is our only option when a vitreous hemorrhage of great magnitude occurs. After a vitrectomy there is often a decent improvement in the vision because we've removed the large, opaque volume of blood that was present between the retina and the outside world.

Since the macula is the most crucial part of the retina, even small changes in its integrity can lead to impaired vision. At any stage of diabetic retinopathy something called clinically significant macular edema (CSME) can occur. Edema is another word for swelling. CSME occurs when diabetes causes fluid to build up in and around the area of the macula causing blurred and distorted vision. CSME often causes the first symptoms of diabetes, as it tends to create a significant shift in nearsightedness. Changes in a person's blood-glucose levels can therefore indirectly lead to a sudden increase in myopia. A sudden, large change in a patient's prescription will often prompt eye doctors to send the patient to the primary care provider for a work up to rule out diabetes before the patient gets new glasses. As the blood-glucose levels fall back within the normal range, the nearsightedness usually subsides. CSME can blur our vision and also distort it by making objects appear smaller or slanted. Swelling in the macula is often treated by a retinal specialist with a focal laser. Since we're dealing with a specific area of the retina, we need a laser that we can aim precisely where we need it to go. We must take great care to relieve the edema in the macula, but not damage the healthy surrounding tissue with the laser. The focal laser is similar to using a scalpel in surgery whereas a PRP laser is more comparable to using a hatchet. Both of these options are greatly effective in achieving the desired result.

Retinal specialists are now using anti-VEGF drugs to stop diabetic retinopathy from destroying vision. These are the same drugs used to treat wet macular degeneration. They are used in the same way, as a series of injections directly into the eye to halt the development of new, abnormal blood vessels caused by the process of neovascularization. Although the drugs are currently used off-label, the results of several small studies suggest that these treatments could become the standard in treating diabetic retinopathy in the future. The term off-label means that the drug is being used in a way that was not indicated when it was approved by the FDA. This is legal and is commonly used in many areas of medicine where the doctor feels that there is reasonable evidence that the specific medicine is helping to treat a patient. Most times, the drug is approved at a later date for the off-label diagnosis in which it was used years before official approval. The anti-VEGF drugs show great promise in the treatment of all neovascular diseases of the eye.

Type II diabetes is a disease that can often be prevented by sticking to some common sense rules of healthy living. The rate of diabetes has increased around the world, but unfortunately it has skyrocketed to levels bordering on epidemic in the United States. In a 2007 study by the National Institute of Health, total medical costs in the U.S. were $116 billion. These were medical costs directly related to diabetes. When we factor in health care costs in which diabetes has played a contributing factor (such as heart disease), the figure rises to an astounding $174 billion—roughly the GDP of the entire country of Ireland! Diabetes affects us as individuals, our families, and the entire health care system of our country. Controlling this disease will take more than medicine. It will take a determined effort on our part to take control of our bodies to improve our well-being and that of society as a whole.

The importance of nutrition and exercise cannot be understated. It is imperative to get 30 minutes of exercise incorporated somewhere into our day. This does not have to mean intense, back-breaking workouts; brisk walking has been shown to be of great value to improving cardio-vascular health. Limiting our intake of sugars and sodium leads to a decreased risk of a long list of health conditions, including diabetes. These are simple adjustments you can make to your life that require only self-discipline to achieve. You will be saving your life and your money in the long run by making smart choices now. Your family will appreciate the effort, too. The most common causes of Type II diabetes are obesity, sedentary lifestyle, smoking and a poor diet. The good news is that all of these causes can be prevented if you have the drive to overcome them.

Hypertension, like diabetes, affects the integrity of blood vessels across our entire body. In the eye it can lead to neovascularization, hemorrhage, stroke and eventual blindness. Hypertension is loosely defined as a blood pressure reading greater than 120/80mmHg. Recently, these numbers have decreased as research indicates that even this figure may be too high. There has also been a pre-hypertensive stage added for people who are at an increased risk for developing true hypertension. High blood pressure is among the leading contributors to death in our country and around the world. It can be a burden on our lives, the lives of our family, and our country's health care network.

Hypertension refers to the increased pressure of the blood flowing through our arteries. The top number (around 120 for a normal pressure reading) is called the systolic reading. This is the pressure in the arteries as the heart contracts and pumps blood throughout the body. As the heart relaxes the pressure is a bit lower and we measure it as the diastolic reading (this is the bottom number, i.e. 80 for a normal measurement). Hypertension is classified into roughly three stages: mild, moderate and severe. When the pressure elevates too high for too long, multiple organ systems are affected. In a similar fashion to diabetes, the kidneys suffer greatly, as the cumulative effects of increased blood pressure flowing through the nephrons of the kidneys eventually take their toll. Hypertension is a leading cause of kidney failure. Blood pressure is routinely measured at health check-ups because of its potential to affect all parts of the body.

The retina is the part of the eye that is most affected by hypertension. The blood vessels that supply the retina are simply smaller branches of arteries and veins that supply blood to the rest of the body. Normally veins and arteries lie in close proximity as they pervade the retina. Veins appear somewhat larger than arteries, but both have a smooth, linear appearance in a person without hypertension. As the blood pressure increases to unhealthy levels, the arteries and veins change shape accordingly. Eye doctors refer to these changes as hypertensive retinopathy, which we divide into three stages: mild, moderate and severe.

Mild hypertensive retinopathy occurs as the arteries begin to narrow. The medical term for this is atherosclerosis. Elevated blood pressure damages the inner wall of the arteries, causing them to constrict. Retinal arteries in a healthy individual are about 2/3 the size of retinal veins. Severe hypertensive retinopathy can reduce the size of the arteries to of the size of the veins. As the retinopathy escalates from mild to moderate, the veins of the retina develop kinks resulting in decreased blood flow. As the condition becomes more severe, retinal veins often take on a "sausage-link" appearance. This is an indication of hypertensive progression in the retina.

Severe hypertension is the stage where symptoms of blurry vision or blindness can surface. In this stage, the blood vessels have been damaged to the point where they begin to leak and hemorrhages are noted throughout the retina. Fatty exudates and cholesterol deposits can also leak from the arteries and deposit throughout the retina. Macular edema occurs as fluid escapes from the blood vessels. We even see swelling of the optic nerve as hypertension worsens. Doctors are paying extra attention for neovascularization to occur at this time as well. These types of changes in the retina indicate that the patient's blood pressure is extremely elevated (often greater than 190/130mmHg), which warrants an immediate visit to the emergency room to reduce the risk of stroke.

When hypertension reaches this level, an eye doctor's greatest fear is an artery or vein occlusion in the eye. The classic symptom of an artery or vein occlusion is a sudden, painless loss of vision in one eye. An interesting point worth repeating is that there is absolutely no pain involved with these blockages even though they are essentially the same as having a stroke in the eye. When we think of having a stroke in any other part of our body we can imagine the paralyzing pain that we experience. In the eye, the blood supply to the retina is cut off and the vision begins to black out, not unlike if you pulled the power cord out of your television. Unfortunately, there is not a whole lot we can do to recover the vision. If one of the small branches of blood vessels is affected, then the vision is usually restored, but when there is a blockage of a large, central vessel, the vision loss is often permanent. These blood vessel occlusions are not only caused by hypertension, but also from blood clots emanating from other parts of the body. If a clot is noted to be the cause of the retinal artery or vein occlusion, then it becomes imperative to locate the source of the clot to prevent other pieces from breaking off and causing a stroke in the brain or heart. For this reason, retinal artery or vein occlusions are considered medical emergencies.

We can clearly see from this chapter that both diabetes and hypertension have the potential to cause blindness. The good news is that the risk of developing these diseases can be greatly reduced for most of us by making the right choices in our lifestyle. Proper diet and exercise will continue to be the most important means for us to keep these diseases in check. The way to ensure that your diet and exercise program is working properly is to have a regular physical exam with your primary care doctor and to have your eyes checked annually by your eye doctor. During an eye exam, you should have your eyes dilated so that your doctor can completely examine the health of your retina as well as your retinal veins and arteries. The eye is the only part of the body where blood vessels can be viewed directly without using a scope or camera. The appearance of the blood vessels in the eye is identical to the way they look in the heart, lungs, kidneys and the rest of the body. When bleeding is noted in the retina from diabetes, you can be certain that it is occurring in all parts of the body. Eye doctors are able to detect diabetes and hypertension simply from a routine eye examination. I personally have seen more than my share of these conditions in previously undiagnosed patients. Indeed, the eyes are the window to the rest of the body.

VISION CORRECTION: FROM GLASSES TO LASIK

The need for better vision became apparent thousands of years ago. The true origin of glasses has been disputed throughout history. Since the production of glass around the time of the Roman Empire, people throughout history realized that changes in the thickness and curvature of glass enhanced their vision. Other properties of glass helped to lead to the development of magnifying glasses. Fish bowls, for example, were known to increase the apparent size of objects when held at the proper distance. Over time glasses evolved and contact lenses developed. Today there is also corrective surgery to enhance vision. In this chapter we'll look at the varieties of ways vision can be improved through corrective measures.

We have already touched briefly on glasses in the second chapter, but it's worth knowing how they have evolved over the years. Bifocals, trifocals and progressive lenses are all ways that we can correct for presbyopia (difficulty seeing up close with our glasses or contacts on) with today's glasses. Bifocals were invented by Benjamin Franklin in 1785. He wanted something that he could wear to state dinners while being able to see other diplomats and his food all with a single pair of glasses. The type of bifocal that Franklin invented is known as an executive bifocal. Essentially there is a line that goes through the center of the lens so that the person looks above the line to see in the distance and below the line to see close up. Over time, Franklin's bifocal evolved into a less conspicuous lens called a flat top bifocal. This is the type of lined bifocal that exists today with a smaller area for viewing near objects. Trifocals emerged when people realized that there is an intermediate distance that remained slightly blurry even when wearing bifocals. Eventually we arrived at the progressive lens which eliminates the lines on the glasses and presents an infinite number of focal points to allow people to see clearly at a distance, close up, and everything in between.

Today, most people are fit into a progressive lens when the need for correction of presbyopia arises. The two main advantages that progressive lenses offer are cosmetic and optical. First, progressive lenses tend to look like any other pair of glasses. This gives people who are self-conscious about their age a great advantage, because no one else will know that the person needs help to see up close unless the wearer tells them. Second, progressive lenses offer an optical advantage because of the infinite number of focal points in the lens. They are called "progressive" lenses because they progressively increase in power from the top to the bottom of the lens. This means that there is a sweet spot in the lens that allows an object to be viewed clearly no matter how far a person is from the object. They are essentially a trifocal without any of the lines in the lens.

Progressive lenses are not perfect. The major disadvantage of a progressive lens is that people have to learn to turn and tilt their head to optimize their vision. The progressive lens has no lines to outline where to look for distance and near. It can take some time to get used to tilting your head to be able to read a book or look at the gauges on your car. Also, due to the nature of the design of the lenses, there are areas of distortion in the far peripheral vision. Instead of predominantly turning your eyes to look at an object in your peripheral vision, you must turn your head. This is a habit that is easier said than done for some people. All in all, once you are used to the progressive lens it is usually preferred over a flat top bifocal.

Today's spectacle lenses are typically made out of plastic. Historically they were made from glass, hence the name "glasses." Glass, however, tends to be very heavy, especially when there is a high amount of prescription in them. "Coke bottle" glasses used to refer to people with high amounts of hyperopia (far-sightedness). The glasses were so thick they resembled the glass bottles that are used to contain soda. Plastic lenses offered lighter weight and thinner spectacle lenses. Polycarbonate lenses are a type of plastic lens that can be made into "high index" lenses to improve the thinness and weight of the glasses. Another advantage of polycarbonate lenses is that they are impact resistant. For this reason, almost all children and athletes have polycarbonate lenses for protection.

The concept of correcting vision without the use of glasses is one that was first thought of hundreds of years ago. In the early 1500's, Leonardo da Vinci designed the first sketches of what we know as contact lenses. Da Vinci was a man of many talents in the fields of art and science. Although he didn't live long enough to see his concept become a reality, it was his idea that inspired the first contact lenses to be produced in the 1880's. The contact lenses of the late 19th century were very different than those of today. They were initially made of glass and covered most of the front of the eye, including the sclera. Glass does not allow much oxygen to penetrate it, so these lenses could only be worn for short periods of time without doing extensive damage to the cornea. Remember, there are no blood vessels in the cornea, so it must obtain oxygen from the air around us. Glass, as you can imagine, also had the disadvantage of being uncomfortable.

As technology progressed, contact lenses went from a glass material to plastic. This is what we refer to today as hard contacts. Unlike previous contact lenses, hard contacts were much smaller. They covered an area slightly smaller than the cornea, which allowed for some oxygen transmission. Hard contact lenses were made out of polymethyl methacrylate (PMMA), a type of plastic. Although hard contact lenses were an improvement over previous generations, they still had two major disadvantages. First, they still didn't allow enough oxygen to reach the cornea. This set up the cornea for an increased risk of scarring (presumably from neovascularization) and infections. Second, there was little room for error to match the fit of the cornea. Frequently, these lenses would pop out of the eye due to a poor fit. Athletes especially had a difficult time with hard contact lenses since they tended to pop out more often during high-impact sports.

In the 1970's, scientists recognized the need for a better contact lens. Rigid Gas Permable (RGP) contacts replaced hard contacts as they provided increased oxygen transmission to the cornea. RGP contact lenses are made out of a silicone and, as the name implies, allow some oxygen to penetrate through the lens to the cornea. The silicone material also provides a better fit so that the contact lens doesn't fall out of the eye as often. RGP contacts have almost completely replaced hard contacts today.

Soon after RGP contacts were made available, soft contact lenses emerged into the market. Soft contact lenses ushered in more oxygen to the cornea while allowing for greater comfort. RGP contacts are still hard enough to change the shape of the cornea, which causes some discomfort. Soft lenses, on the other hand, drape over the cornea to allow for an enormous difference in comfort. If you imagine your cornea as a sponge, RGP contacts fit over it like a cereal bowl. The sponge gets contorted to fit within the bowl. Alternatively, soft contacts would rest over top of the sponge like a blanket. They don't affect the soft tissue of the cornea and thus are more comfortable.

Soft contact lenses are far more common today than RGP lenses, in part because technology has rendered them healthy, comfortable and affordable. Today's soft contact lenses are available in three modalities: one month, two week and one day disposable lenses. Disposing of the contacts frequently decreases the risk of infection and inflammatory conditions. In 2000, the latest generation of soft contact lenses emerged offering the highest oxygen transmission yet. The lenses are made out of a silicone hydrogel material. The latest generation of lenses allows enough oxygen to reach the cornea that many of them have been FDA approved to wear on the eye for 30 continuous days and nights. Many of the new contact lenses on the market today allow greater comfort than previous generations due to their increased ability to stay moist over a longer period of the day.

Until relatively recently, anyone with a moderate amount of astigmatism had to wear RGP contact lenses to correct their vision. Now, toric contact lenses can correct for nearly any amount of astigmatism. We can now fit new patients with more comfortable soft lenses where we lacked this technology in the 1980's. Toric contact lenses work by adding a small prism to the contact lens to act as a weight. Remember that astigmatism means that the cornea is more oval shaped, so any contact lens placed on the eye must be able to stay in one position to correct one's vision. Any rotation would cause the vision to be distorted as if you were to twist your glasses 90 degrees. Gravity pulls the weight to the correct position on the eye. For this reason, if you wear toric contact lenses and lay on your side for a while, the lenses may rotate and cause a bit of blurry vision until they finally settle in place.

There are several options for those who don't have arms long enough to read a book with contact lenses in place. First, you could put reading glasses on over the contact lenses. This will give you the best vision for reading and distance vision. Unfortunately, you won't be able to read and look in the distance without removing the glasses. This option can be cumbersome, because you must take the glasses on and off frequently. Also, most people wear contact lenses because they prefer not to wear glasses. Another option would be a monovision fit with contact lenses. Here, we fit one eye with a distance prescription and the other eye with a near prescription. This allows people to see at all distances at the same time. As you can imagine, it does take a few days to get your eyes and brain used to this sort of vision, but for many people it is a fantastic way of getting around without the need for reading glasses. Monovision correction greatly reduces one's depth perception making it less than ideal for everyone. Golfers and tennis players for example, tend to have a difficult time judging the distance of the ball, which can wreak havoc on their game.

Multifocal contact lenses offer a third option for people who are dealing with the joys of presbyopia. Unlike monovision, where each eye is completely dedicated to either distance or near vision, multifocal lenses allow each eye to be able to focus at both far and near objects. This technology provides the advantage of increased depth perception. For the most part, multifocal contacts lenses allow for better optics due to the dual nature of distance and near vision in each eye. Most multifocal contact lenses work by having a small area of distance vision in the center of the lens surrounded by a ring of near vision along the outer edge. It's similar to a bull's eye with the center circle containing correction for distance vision and an outer ring correcting for the near vision. In this way, it doesn't really matter if the lens rotates much, because there will always be a near area to see through. The main disadvantage of multifocal lenses is the size of the lens itself. Since they sit directly on the cornea they are relatively small, and the same prescription in one's bifocal glasses must be transferred into a tiny contact lens. This accounts for many of the complaints of halos or a glow around objects when viewed through these contact lenses. For many people, however, this is a small price to pay to be able to have decent vision without the need for glasses.

Contact lenses not only improve vision, but are also used in a variety of other ways. Colored contact lenses can be used for cosmetic purposes to change the appearance of the iris. Sometimes colored contacts are used for a more serious purpose, such as to mask a defect in the iris. A coloboma is a hole or missing piece of the eye that usually results from a congenital birth defect. An iris coloboma, for example, occurs when a part of the iris is missing causing a misshapen pupil to form. This pie wedge shaped part that is absent almost always occurs on the bottom area of the iris, from about four to seven o'clock on a clock dial. The misshaped pupil can cause light sensitivity and a double image to form on the retina causing blurry vision. A special colored contact lens is often placed on the affected eye to create a rounder pupil. This improves the vision and also the appearance of the eye. These contact lenses can be specially made to exactly match the person's original eye color.

Contact lenses often play a role in the treatment of eye injuries. Corneal abrasions tend to be one of the more common eye injuries in the emergency room. Abrasions can occur from a wide variety of reasons, such as rubbing the eye too hard, taking a tennis ball to the eye, being poked by a tree branch, etc. The tiniest scratch can cause debilitating pain. This is because the cornea is the most innervated part of the body. There are no blood vessels in the cornea, but if you've ever had a corneal abrasion, you know there are plenty of nerve endings! Fortunately, the cornea heals quite rapidly. Small abrasions will often heal on their own with some lubricating or antibiotic eye drops. For larger abrasions, however, we often use a contact lens to facilitate the healing process. A corneal abrasion is similar to a scrape on the skin of your arm that you may get if you've fallen off of a bicycle. When the wound is open, it can get very irritated and uncomfortable if you rub it with your hand. Each time we blink, our eyelids rub across the surface of the cornea and due to the large concentration of nerve endings it results in a lot of pain when we have a large abrasion. We sometimes place a contact lens on the eye to act as a bandage and reduce the mechanical friction of the eyelid rubbing on the cornea. The contact lens also allows the top layer of the cornea to anchor itself to the rest of the cornea while healing, which is important with larger abrasions to prevent the abrasion from reoccurring. Patients certainly appreciate the relief that a contact lens can bring to a scratched cornea.

Another interesting application of contact lenses is in the field of orthokeratology. This idea came about when doctors realized that when hard contact lenses were placed on the eye for a period of time, they seemed to change the vision temporarily after they were removed. People who were nearsighted, for example, could see fairly well after removing their contacts for a short time. As we discovered earlier, the cornea is a very soft tissue that will conform to the shape of hard contacts. Orthokeratology evolved as doctors realized that they could manipulate the shape and curvature of the contact lens to mold the cornea into the proper shape to eliminate myopia. In this technique, the person is fitted for a hard contact lens that is specifically designed to make the cornea flatter to correct for nearsightedness or steeper to correct for farsightedness. The person inserts the contact lenses into the eyes just before bedtime. Over the course of seven to eight hours the contacts gently reshape the cornea so that when the contacts are removed in the morning, the vision is as clear as it would be with glasses or contacts. The vision gradually worsens throughout the day as the cornea expands back to its natural shape. For most of the day though, people can experience clear vision without the need for glasses or contact lenses.

Orthokeratology can be used in many applications. We use it for swimmers who need vision correction, but cannot wear soft contact lenses for swimming. People with small amounts of myopia do well with this method because their vision tends to stay clear for a longer period of time compared to folks with greater amounts of myopia. Finally, people with eyes that are too dry to wear contacts during the day benefit from wearing contacts at night, since they can rest their eyes rather than having them dry out during the work day. This is a great benefit for those who have run out of options for vision correction.

There are limits to the benefits orthokeratology can provide. The biggest drawback is that it can only be used to treat mild amounts of myopia, hyperopia and astigmatism. Also, as the prescription increases, the length of time that one can expect decent vision decreases. Someone with moderate amounts of myopia, for example, may only have six to eight hours before the vision begins to revert back to its uncorrected form. Another downside to this method of vision correction is that the contact lenses tend to be slightly uncomfortable for a few weeks until the person gets used to wearing them. Since they have to be inserted overnight, some folks find it difficult to sleep with the contacts at first until they become accustomed to the fit of the lens on their eye. Drawbacks aside, orthokeratology is an innovative method of vision correction that came about with the advancement in the technology of contact lenses.

The most recent breakthrough in vision correction came in the mid 1990's with the FDA approval of laser vision correction. For the first time in history we have a method of correcting our vision without the need to wear corrective lenses. Prior to lasers being used to eliminate our glasses and contacts, a procedure called radial keratotomy (RK) was being done in an attempt to alter the shape of the cornea and thus improve distance vision. RK involves a surgeon using a blade to make carefully calculated incisions in the cornea to correct for small to moderate amounts of myopia. During the 1980's thousands of these procedures were helping people to see without the need for corrective lenses. There were several drawbacks to RK that made it less than ideal. First, the benefits of the procedure tended not to last very long. Only about half of the people who received RK had 20/20 vision after 10 years. Many even needed corrective lenses again to maintain the quality of vision that they had just after surgery. Second, each eye had to be done roughly six weeks apart to facilitate healing. This lengthened the vision correction process to about two months by the time both eyes had the procedure. Finally, RK tended to create a lot of glare in the vision after surgery. Halos around lights made night vision especially troubling. The incorporation of the laser eliminated many of the nuances of refractive surgery.

Photorefractive keratectomy (PRK) gained FDA approval in the mid-1990's as the first use of a laser to correct refractive error. PRK can correct very high amounts of myopia (around -12.00D), hyperopia (about +4.00D) and astigmatism (roughly 4.00D). A type of laser called an excimer laser is used to reshape the front surface of the cornea. Remember that people with myopia (nearsightedness) tend to have a longer or steeper curve to their cornea than normal. The goal of laser vision correction is to shorten or flatten out this curve at the center of the cornea to the point where light entering through the cornea will project onto the perfect point of the retina for us to have clear vision. In people with hyperopia (farsightedness), the opposite is true. Here, the outer portion of the cornea is manipulated by the laser to give a steeper central cornea, thus changing the focal point on the retina. The use of the laser allows the surgeon to make precise maneuvers in order to get the desired shape of the cornea.

PRK is still used today and works well for many people, but it is not without drawbacks. First, PRK takes some time for the vision to reach its full potential. As we mentioned earlier, a laser is being used to reshape the front surface of the eye. The result of this is a properly shaped cornea, but essentially a corneal abrasion is formed. The vision can be blurry until the cornea can completely heal its front surface, which can take weeks to months. Second, there is usually some discomfort associated with PRK as the healing process occurs. The pain is usually mild to moderate and tends to last only a few days. On occasion a contact lens is placed over the cornea to facilitate the healing process and reduce the amount of discomfort after surgery.

The advantage of PRK is that it can be done on relatively thin corneas. Laser vision correcting procedures require various amounts of tissue to reshape the cornea. It is not unlike a clay sculpture. An artist needs enough clay to work with depending on the size and detail of the final piece of art. The same is true in laser surgery; the greater the amount of myopia, hyperopia or astigmatism, the more the corneal tissue will need to be manipulated into the proper form to produce the desired result. Someone with -7.00D of myopia, for example, will need to have a thicker cornea to be a good candidate for surgery than someone with -1.50D of myopia. The reason PRK can be done on a thinner cornea than other laser procedures is because it does not require the formation of a flap to do the surgery. We will discuss this further in a moment.

In the late 1990's, LASIK was approved by the FDA and has been the most popular form of laser vision correcting procedures. LASIK stands for Laser-Assisted In-Situ Keratomileusis. It can correct large amounts of hyperopia, myopia and astigmatism, although slightly less than that of PRK. The principle is the same as PRK in that the front surface of the cornea is reshaped; however, the surgical procedure is different. LASIK first involves a laser scan of the front surface of the eye to determine precise measurements and curvature readings of the cornea so the vision can be fully corrected. Once this is done, a laser is used to create a very thin flap of tissue from the outer layer of the cornea. The creation of a corneal flap is what makes LASIK unique. The flap is gently moved aside while the laser resurfaces the exposed surface of the cornea to the exact specifications needed to correct one's vision. The flap is then replaced over the cornea. There are no stitches required, since the incision created by the laser is so thin that the corneal tissue is able to heal completely on its own. The corneal flap acts as a bandage so that there is very little discomfort as the cornea continues to heal. The reshaping of the cornea takes place just underneath the outer layer of the cornea, so the vision tends to be fairly clear immediately after surgery. Compared to PRK, the initial vision after LASIK is much improved.

The corneal flap created in LASIK has both benefits and drawbacks. The flap allows the cornea to heal comfortably and vision tends to be sharper in a shorter amount of time. The downside of creating a flap in the cornea is that it requires a thicker cornea to correct the vision. Since some of the corneal thickness is used to create the flap, we cannot correct as much myopia, hyperopia or astigmatism with LASIK as we can with PRK. Some members of the military, in particularly Rangers and those who jump out of planes at high altitudes, are required to undergo PRK rather than LASIK due to the uncertainty of the flap separating from the cornea under combat conditions.

If one's prescription is too great relative to the amount of corneal thickness, then laser vision correction is no longer an option. For these people, the best surgical option is to have a lens implanted in the small space between the iris and the natural lens. These lenses are referred to as Implantable Collamer Lenses (ICL). While this procedure usually sounds pretty scary when I first mention it to people, it's actually painless and has produced many happy patients. It is like inserting a contact lens in your eye rather than on your eye. The ICL is made out of a biocompatible plastic that is customized to the exact prescription of the eye. Two small incisions are made in the cornea to create a channel to slip the ICL through. The ICL is tightly folded and placed through the incisions, and is unfolded when it is in the proper placement just behind the iris. This is similar to the procedure that is used to insert an artificial lens in the eye during cataract surgery. A benefit of the ICL is that it can be removed very easily if the vision changes at all after the procedure. It can also be used to correct up to 16D of myopia and low to moderate amounts of astigmatism. Since this procedure was FDA approved in 2005, thousands of people have enjoyed the outstanding vision that the ICL can provide to those who are unable to undergo laser vision correction.

As we've learned from this chapter, vision correction has come a long way since it was first discovered that glass can be used to enhance vision. In the future, contact lens technology will continue to progress, especially in the area of multifocal contact lenses. You can expect better optics and increased comfort as companies strive to produce a contact that can be tolerable to everyone. Surgical vision correction is sure to improve as well. As ICL technology improves, you can expect an increase in the number of patients undergoing this procedure and a decrease in its cost. Similarly, laser vision correction will not be going away any time soon. As long as people continue to suffer from blurry vision, new and improved ways of correction will continue to progress.

CONCLUSION

"The eyes are the window to the soul." This famous saying is not far from the truth. The eyes are indeed an indicator of the overall health of our body. Nearly every systemic condition can manifest itself in the eyes. Diabetes and hypertension are the two that grab the most headlines, but cancer, Lyme disease, arthritis and multiple sclerosis can all display warning signs in the eyes as they lurk in the body. It is for this reason that an annual eye exam is so important. In medicine, there is a general rule that the earlier a condition is detected, the better the chance of a positive prognosis.

Our eyes are also important for our survival. They alert us when danger appears in our environment. They indicate which foods are more appealing to eat. They also relay information to the brain about the body language of others around us. In fact, our eyes are involved in nearly every decision we make. It's no wonder that our vision is regarded as the most important of our five senses.

In this book we only touched the surface of the major aspects of eye care; the scope of optometry is too broad to be covered in this book. There are many other fascinating areas of optometry, such as vision therapy, that can be used to treat amblyopia (lazy eye); low vision materials like magnifiers and zoom lenses that can assist those affected by macular degeneration and glaucoma; and future technology such as contacts that contain chips to guide our soldiers in battle or deliver time-released medicine to glaucoma patients. It is my hope that this book has armed you with the knowledge to further pursue these and other areas of eye care in which you have an interest. I would encourage you to ask questions to your eye care provider if something isn't clear. Ask about the most recent treatment or new technology of an eye disease or procedure. The patient who is involved in his or her own health care will be much better off than those who lack an understanding. Forming a relationship with your health provider will improve your own health and medicine as a whole.

Glossary

Amblyopia: Medical term for "lazy eye". Amblyopia means that the vision cannot be corrected to 20/20 in one or both eyes. There are several causes of amblyopia.

Astigmatism: A curvature of the cornea or lens in the eye that causes distorted vision.

Cataract: A clouding or opacity of the lens.

Cone Cells: Located in the macula of the retina. Cone cells allow us to see fine detail in our vision.

Conjunctiva: Clear membrane covering the front of the eye and inner eyelids. This tissue primarily gets inflamed during an episode of "pink eye".

Cornea: The clear, dome-shaped cap in the front of the eye. The cornea is responsible for proper focusing of incoming light rays on our retina.

Drusen: By-product of cellular waste that accumulates in the macula. Drusen lead to vision loss in macular degeneration.

Glaucoma: Progressive damage to the optic nerve over time. This disease has a wide range of causes and clinical presentations.

Hyperopia: Medical term for farsightedness. A person with hyperopia generally has better vision when looking in the distance rather than looking at near.

Iris: The colored part in the front of the eye. The iris contracts and expands, forming the pupil size depending on the illumination of our surroundings.

Keratoconus: Disease of the eye in which the cornea becomes progressively thin and cone shaped. People suffering from keratoconus often experience blurred vision due to astigmatism.

LASIK: Acronym for Laser Assisted In Situ Keratomileusis. LASIK is a vision correcting procedure for the treatment of myopia, hyperopia and astigmatism.

Lens: Located directly behind the iris. The lens works with the cornea to properly focus images on our retina. The lens allows us to quickly change our focus from objects at near to distance.

Macula: The center of the retina. This is where most of the fine detail in our vision is detected.

Myopia: Medical term for nearsightedness. When a person has myopia, they need visual correction for improved distance vision.

Neovascularization: The process by which the body forms new blood vessels in response to decreased oxygen and nutrient supply. The problem with these new blood vessels is that they are extremely fragile and inevitably break, causing hemorrhaging and scarring. Neovascularization can occur in glaucoma, diabetes and macular degeneration.

Ophthalmologist: An eye doctor who diagnoses, treats and manages diseases and conditions of the eye. Ophthalmologists are surgeons who generally specialize in a particular area of eye care, such as the cornea, retina or neurological conditions.

Optician: A person who dispenses and cuts glasses.

Optic Nerve: Nerve that connects the eye to the brain. This nerve transmits the signal from the retina to the brain.

Optometrist: An eye doctor who examines, diagnoses, treats and manages diseases and disorders of the eye and visual system. Optometrists provide the same care as ophthalmologists, except that they do not perform major surgery.

Presbyopia: Visual phenomenon that occurs primarily for people in their late 30's or early 40's in which it becomes difficult to focus on near objects.

Progressive Lens: An eyeglass lens that allows us to see at distance, near and everything in between. Progressive lenses differ from trifocals in that they do not have lines in them.

PRK: Acronym for photorefractive keratectomy. This is a laser vision correcting procedure that is similar to LASIK except there is no flap made on the cornea. This procedure is the treatment of choice for vision correction when LASIK is unavailable.

Retina: The inside rear portion of the eye that detects and transmits signals to the brain to form an image. The retina is made of rod and cone cells, and contains a rich network of blood vessels to provide the many nutrients it needs to function.

Rod Cells: Located in the retina. Rods allow us to see in dimly illuminated environments.

Sclera: White, outer portion of the eye. The sclera is thick to provide protection to the eye.

Vitreous: Gel-like substance found in the globe of the eye. The vitreous is clear to allow light to pass through to the retina.

Index

CPSIA information can be obtained at www.ICGtesting.com
Printed in the USA
LVOW051946140413

329067LV00004B/29/P